STRENGTHENING POST-EBOLA HEALTH SYSTEMS

STRENGTHENING POST-EBOLA HEALTH SYSTEMS

From Response to Resilience in Guinea, Liberia, and Sierra Leone

Ramesh Govindaraj, Christopher H. Herbst,
and John Paul Clark, Editors

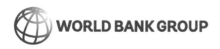 **WORLD BANK GROUP**

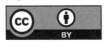
This study was undertaken in 2015–16. Its findings, recommendations, and conclusions reflect a contemporaneous understanding of the situation in Guinea, Liberia, and Sierra Leone at the time, and must be read as such. Several welcome public health initiatives have since been launched by the countries themselves, as well as by development partners, and more refined and in-depth data have become available. All these will necessarily have a bearing on the prospects for pandemic preparedness and health systems strengthening in these three countries. However, the authors believe that the broad conclusions of this study still hold, and the policy choices and program priorities highlighted here continue to be relevant to the three countries and beyond.

Contents

Boxes

Figures

Tables

Preface

The 2013–16 Ebola Virus Disease (EVD) outbreak in West Africa, which caused a major loss of life and socioeconomic disruption in the region—particularly in the countries of Guinea, Liberia, and Sierra Leone—was the most widespread outbreak of the disease in history. In support of country governments, the World Bank played a key role in the global response effort, drawing on its ability to mobilize financing and technical knowledge, and to leverage its close working relationships with ministries, United Nations agencies and other development partners, civil society, and the private sector.

The crisis has demonstrated, at a very high human, social, and economic cost, the imperative of investing in effective and efficient health systems and establishing public health and disease surveillance systems as a priority public regional good. With the end of that Ebola outbreak, the World Bank's engagement in Guinea, Liberia, and Sierra Leone shifted from a response effort toward a focus on rebuilding and strengthening the very foundations of health systems that were already weak prior to the crisis.

Initiated while Ebola was still raging in the three most-affected countries in West Africa, and produced in close collaboration with our academic and development partners, this report reflects on the challenge of strengthening health systems in the three countries, and how to move beyond just getting the number of Ebola cases to zero. Within the context of limited fiscal space, and emphasizing the particular need to strengthen health workforce capacity and regional disease surveillance systems, the report discusses some of the opportunities and options to help create viable, resilient, and fiscally sustainable health systems in Guinea, Liberia, and Sierra Leone.

In the absence of a massive, well-organized global response, the devastating Ebola virus epidemic could have become a global catastrophe. The same commitment is now needed to help rebuild and strengthen the health system in each of the three countries and beyond. The news in mid-May of 2017 of another Ebola episode in the Democratic Republic of Congo reminds us that such an effort continues to be a particularly important and urgent priority. I hope that this report is beneficial to policy makers and practitioners working on health-system strengthening in the Sub-Saharan Africa region and elsewhere, and that it can inform better preparedness, resilience, and prosperity for our clients.

Olusoji Adeyi
Director, Health, Nutrition, and
Population Global Practice
The World Bank

Acknowledgments

This report was prepared at the request, and under the overall leadership, of Makhtar Diop, World Bank Vice President for the Africa Region, and it benefited from the guidance provided by Lynne D. Sherburne-Benz, Senior Regional Advisor in the Africa Regional Vice Presidency.

The overall report was led by Ramesh Govindaraj, Lead Specialist, Health, Nutrition, and Population, Christopher H. Herbst, Senior Health Specialist, and John Paul Clark, Senior Health Specialist. Erika Lutz, Senior Nutrition Specialist, provided critical support on chapter 1. Christopher Rockmore, Senior Economist, led chapter 2 and sections on the Investment Plan and the Fiscal Space Analysis. Christopher H. Herbst, Senior Health Specialist, led chapter 3 and sections on Human Resources for Health. John Paul Clark, Senior Health Specialist, led chapter 4 and sections on Disease Surveillance. General guidance was provided by Trina Haque, Practice Manager, Olusoji Adeyi, Director, and Timothy G. Evans, Senior Director, of the Health, Nutrition, and Population Global Practice.

The report was written jointly by a team drawn from the World Bank's Health, Nutrition, and Population Global Practice, academia, and partner organizations. The writing team of the Health Systems and Financing sections consisted of Ramesh Govindaraj, Moulay Driss Zine Eddine El Idrissi, Christopher Rockmore, and Netsanent Walelign (all of the World Bank). The writing team of the health workforce chapter and sections consisted of Laurence Codjia (World Health Organization [WHO]), Prarthna Dayal (Nossal Institute of Global Health, University of Melbourne), Matt Edwards (Center for Workforce Intelligence [CfWI], UK), John Fellows (CfWI), Alex Gasasira (WHO Liberia), Christopher H. Herbst (World Bank), Robert Marten (WHO Sierra Leone), Barbara McPake (Nossal Institute), Cristina Sanchez (CfWI), Barbara Tomai (CfWI), and Tana Wuliji (WHO). The writing team of the disease surveillance chapter and sections was Oluwayemisi Busola Ajumobi and John Paul Clark (both of the World Bank).

The team benefited immensely from extensive country consultations, consultations with partner agencies, including the WHO, UNICEF and the U.S. Centers for Disease Control and Prevention, the inputs and close collaboration of country task team leaders Ibrahim Magazi (Guinea), Rianna Mohammed and Shunsuke Mabuchi (Liberia), and Francisca Ayodeji Akala (Sierra Leone), as well as the feedback from the relevant country economists from the World Bank's Macroeconomics and Fiscal Management Global Practice. The team also benefited from guidance and comments received from Pierre Laporte (Country Director for Guinea) and Rachidi Radji (Country Manager, Guinea), Henry Kerali (Country Director for Ghana, Liberia, and Sierra Leone), Rachid Benmessaoud (Country Director for Nigeria), as well as the respective country management units. The thoughtful review comments from Mickey Chopra, Christoph Kurowski, Akiko Maeda, and Patrick Osewe (all of the World Bank's Health, Nutrition and Population Global Practice) were very useful in finalizing the study. The comments received from the participants at the Special Session on Ebola Response at the World Bank's Spring Meetings in 2015, where the initial findings of the study were presented, are also acknowledged. Finally, the authors are grateful for the careful review and comments from Punam Chuhan-Pole, Lead Economist, and the team of the Chief Economist's Office for the Africa Region.

The financial support from the Health Financing, Service Delivery, and Healthy Societies Global Solutions Groups of the World Bank for the publication of this study is gratefully acknowledged. Also acknowledged is the financial support from the State and Peacebuilding Fund, which supported the health workforce analyses.

The State and Peacebuilding Fund is a global fund to finance critical development operations and analysis in situations of fragility, conflict, and violence. The State and Peacebuilding Fund is kindly supported by Australia, Denmark, Germany, The Netherlands, Norway, Sweden, The United Kingdom, and the World Bank.

Abbreviations

AfDB	African Development Bank
ATS	agents technique de santé
BPEHS	Basic Package of Essential Health Services
CDC	U.S. Centers for Disease Control and Prevention
CFSVA	Comprehensive Food Security & Vulnerability Analysis
CHW	community health worker
CHV	community health volunteer
DSR	disease surveillance and response
EAIDSNet	East Africa Infectious Disease Surveillance Network
EMS	Event Management System
EU	European Union
EVD	Ebola virus disease
EWARN	Early Warning and Response Network
FAO	Food and Agriculture Organization (of the UN)
GLEWS	Global Early Warning System
GOARN	Global Outbreak Alert Response Network (of the WHO)
HMIS	Health Management Information Systems
HRH	human resources for health
ICT	information and communication technology
IDA	International Development Association
IDSR	Integrated Disease Surveillance and Response
IHR	International Health Regulations
IMF	International Monetary Fund
MBB	Marginal Bottlenecks Budgeting
MBDS	Mekong Basin Disease Surveillance
MBRTs	multisectoral border response teams
MECIDS	Middle East Consortium for Infectious Disease Surveillance
MTEF	Medium-Term Expenditure Framework

NGO	nongovernmental organization
OECD	Organisation for Economic Co-operation and Development
OIE	World Organization for Animal Health
PBF	performance-based financing
PFM	public financial management
PPE	personal protective equipment
PPHSN	Pacific Public Health Surveillance Network
RDSR	regional disease surveillance and response
REDISSE	Regional Disease Surveillance Systems Enhancement
SACIDS	Southern Africa Consortium for Infectious Disease Surveillance
SARS	severe acute respiratory syndrome
THE	total health expenditures
UHC	universal health coverage
UN	United Nations
UNICEF	United Nations Children's Fund
WBG	World Bank Group
WHO	World Health Organization

All dollar amounts are U.S. dollars unless specified otherwise.

CHAPTER 1

Introduction and Context

The Ebola virus disease (EVD) outbreak in parts of West Africa—which particularly affected Guinea, Liberia, and Sierra Leone and peaked in August–September 2014—demonstrated, at very high human, social, and economic cost, the imperative of investing in health systems and establishing public health surveillance and preparedness systems as a priority global public good. The impact of this outbreak was felt well beyond the health sector: Entire economies were severely affected, food became scarce, schools were shut down, and overall development efforts stalled. The rapid spread of the disease in the context of weak health systems set back health, nutrition, and socioeconomic gains made over the past decade. In economic terms, the World Bank estimates that, in 2015 alone, the three most-affected countries (Guinea, Liberia, and Sierra Leone) lost US$2 billion in forgone economic growth because of the EVD outbreak, while the broader region of West Africa lost as much as US$30 billion.

The EVD outbreak and health systems recovery process occurred within a challenging socioeconomic context. Guinea is one of the poorest countries in the world, ranking 178 out of 187 countries on the United Nations Development Programme's Human Development Index, just behind Liberia at 174 and Sierra Leone at 177. Gross national income (GNI) per capita (Guinea: US$440; Liberia: US$370; Sierra Leone: US$700) and other socioeconomic indicators have crept up in the past few years, but remain discouragingly low. The health systems in the three countries were extremely weak, and the health and nutrition outcomes were poor, even prior to the EVD crisis, and this situation was further exacerbated by the EVD crisis. Continuing to rebuild and strengthen the health systems in these countries is therefore a priority.

Goal and Scope of the Post-Ebola Study

Despite the tremendous challenges and the human suffering that Ebola has caused in Guinea, Liberia, and Sierra Leone, the EVD crisis also presents opportunities to strengthen health systems in these affected countries. Media and international development interest have been high. Technical support and financial resources have surged in these countries, creating a window of opportunity for reinforced action on health systems strengthening. This study, initiated while Ebola was still raging in all three most-affected countries, addresses the challenge of enabling the development of viable, resilient, and fiscally sustainable health systems in those countries to go beyond just getting the number of Ebola cases to zero.

The study takes the proceedings of a high-level meeting with key global public health stakeholders—convened at the WHO in Geneva on December 10–11, 2014—to discuss and identify the priority areas for building resilient health systems in the Ebola-affected countries.[1] At the meeting, the most critical issues for public health resilience and emergency preparedness were identified as (1) adequate fiscal space, (2) an effective health workforce, and (3) continuous disease surveillance; these are the three areas examined in this study.

The overall goal of this study is thus twofold:

1. To assess the capacity of the health systems of the three most-affected countries in terms of their ability to deliver quality health services to their populations, to perform core public health functions on a routine basis, and to respond to public health emergencies; and

2. To identify the highest-impact strategies to help these countries to strengthen their health systems to be more effective and resilient, drilling down into three key aspects of the health system; that is, fiscal space for universal health coverage (UHC), development and deployment of an effective health workforce, and continuous disease surveillance.[2]

The lessons from this analysis are expected to contribute not only to efforts to rebuild the health systems of Guinea, Liberia, and Sierra Leone, but also to highlight issues that are likely to be of critical relevance for strengthening health systems in other low-income countries in Sub-Saharan Africa.

The findings, recommendations, and conclusions in the report reflect a contemporary understanding of the realities at the country level at the time the study was undertaken in 2015–16, recognition of dire and widespread needs, reasonable estimates of financial resources from domestic and international sources in the medium term, and the plausible effects of the implementation capacity during the same period. They are subject to change as more complete data become available, and as the countries and development partners learn from the implementation of the many initiatives launched since this study was initiated. To that extent, the report is indicative rather than definitive, and is meant to inform policy choices and program priorities.

Structure of This Synthesis Report

This report is structured around the three key areas identified as the most critical for establishing resilient health systems in Guinea, Liberia, and Sierra Leone: fiscal space, health workforce, and disease surveillance. Chapter 2 considers the issue of fiscal space. It takes a comparative perspective to review and assess, vis-a-vis WHO's health systems building blocks framework, the post-Ebola national health systems' investment plans prepared by the three countries, including assessments of the proposed outputs, cost estimates, and financing gaps. It then evaluates the available and potential resources for their implementation in the fiscal space section. Chapter 3 examines the adequacy of the health workforce for each country. It assesses the extent to which their national investment plans are appropriate in meeting human resources for health (HRH) needs and goals, discusses the cost and financing implications of achieving various targets, and provides key recommendations on moving forward. Chapter 4 discusses the imperative of developing an effective national and cross-national disease surveillance and response network in the region, as well as the technical and cost implications of such a network for each of the three countries. Chapter 5 wraps up the report with key conclusions and recommendations.

The key findings of each chapter are summarized below.

Chapter 2: National Investment Plans and Fiscal Space Analysis
Although the scope and reach of the investment plans in Guinea, Liberia, and Sierra Leone vary, given their different needs, contexts, and available resources, all the plans include relevant initiatives to strengthen the six essential building blocks of effective health systems proposed by the WHO in 2007.[3] The baseline, medium, and aggressive costing scenarios proposed by each country represent a recognition of the fact that the extent to which the health systems in each country can be strengthened is contingent on the quantum of resources that might be available. Viewed in terms of health spending per capita, the costs associated with the proposed health plans are reasonable, even when compared with average health expenditures in Sub-Saharan Africa. The key, though, will be the

efficient and effective translation of the investment plans into operational plans that are then implemented.

Although governments must leverage domestic resources to finance their health system investment plans, sustained international support will be necessary to ensure that the baseline scenarios can be implemented. The main sources of increased fiscal space through domestic resources are improved efficiency in the allocation and use of health sector resources, as well as a movement away from a reliance on direct, out-of-pocket payments to combinations of pooling and prepayment mechanisms, with varying degrees of financing from general revenues to promote universal health coverage. The countries should also work with the International Monetary Fund (IMF) to see if a relaxation of the deficit financing ceilings they currently face may be possible (at least for the short to medium term) so that the overall allocations to the health and related social sectors can be increased.

Chapter 3: Plans to Scale up and Improve the Distribution of the Health Work Force

To address prevailing needs within a constrained fiscal space scenario, a paradigm shift in who to train and how to train health workers is needed in all three countries. The primary focus should be on strategies to scale up the rural health workforce—this is where the majority of the population lives and capacity constraints are greatest. While the strengthening of competencies for UHC can be delivered through innovative and supportive short-term strategies, promising medium- and longer-term approaches include so-called rural pipeline policies, which focus on producing cost-effective and high-impact lower and mid-level health workers with profiles more amenable to working in rural areas. Ultimately, all three countries must recognize the need to carry out comprehensive health labor market assessments to guide the specific interventions needed to produce a fit-for-purpose health workforce.

Chapter 4: Scaling Up the Disease Surveillance System

Improved collaboration among countries in the form of a regional disease surveillance network is a critical step that will require strengthening cross-sectoral capacity as well as regional cooperation to detect earlier, better prepare, and rapidly respond to infectious disease threats at the animal-human-ecosystem interface. This is an economically sound investment and a practical way to leverage domestic and international resources to greater effect.

Chapter 5: Overall Conclusions and Recommendations

Taken together, the three issues addressed in this post-Ebola report provide compelling evidence that Guinea, Liberia, and Sierra Leone, working closely with the international community, have a historic opportunity to act in a manner that will go some distance toward mitigating the risks of enormous human, social, and economic consequences in the event of future outbreaks of disease. At the same time, acting on the recommendations put forward in this study should strengthen these countries' health systems and ensure a reasonable level of coverage and quality of health care services. The recommendations can also inform policy discussions in other developing countries that face similar constraints, risks, and trade-offs.

Notes

1. The high-level meeting was held at the WHO in Geneva to discuss and identify the priority areas for building resilient health systems in the Ebola-affected countries, December 10–11, 2014. http://www.who.int/healthsystems/ebola/meeting10122014/en/.
2. The chapters on human resources for health (HRH) and on disease surveillance in this synthesis report benefited greatly from a collaboration with the WHO and with the U.S. Centers for Disease Control and Prevention (CDC), respectively, among others.
3. The 2007 WHO framework includes six building blocks of health systems (1) service delivery; (2) health workforce; (3) information; (4) medical products, vaccines, and technologies; (5) financing; and (6) governance (stewardship) http://www.who.int/healthsystems/strategy/everybodys_business.pdf.

References

GHRF (Global Health Risk Framework for the Future) Commission. 2016. *The Neglected Dimension of Global Security: A Framework to Counter Infectious Disease Crises*. Washington, DC: National Academies Press.

WHO (World Health Organization). 2005. *International Health Regulations*, 3rd ed. http://www.who.int/ihr/publications/9789241580496/en/

CHAPTER 2

National Investment Plans and Fiscal Space Analysis

Introduction

This chapter reviews the investment plans, costs, and fiscal space for the three countries. The discussion of the investment plans covers the approach and methods used in the plans and an assessment of their content relative to the WHO's definition of the six essential building blocks of health systems strengthening. The cost of the plans is assessed relative to existing resources and capacity to execute the work. Finally, the fiscal space analysis reviews the current situation and possible sources of additional resources.

Process of Developing the Health Systems Strengthening Investment Plans

Recognizing the need for country-level coordination and planning, as the Ebola virus disease (EVD) crisis started to recede, each of the three Ebola-affected countries developed—through a consultative process—a national post-Ebola health systems strengthening investment plan. These plans—prepared with strong government leadership, the involvement of relevant stakeholders, and support from the international community—outline key proposed investments that need to be made in health systems strengthening. Although the international community played a supportive role, the scenarios outlined by each country in its investment plan were very much the outcome of negotiations among domestic stakeholders and were determined by the political economy of each country.

Beyond providing technical assistance, along with the WHO and other partners, the World Bank Group also helped to evaluate the fiscal space in each country. The fiscal space analysis, which is covered later in this chapter, connects the funding requirements to the known, possible, and potential resources of the countries. This was a key input into the development of the final plans.

The national investment plans all address the various aspects of health systems, but have different visions of how to achieve a resilient health care system. Whereas Guinea and Liberia stress the broader overall objective of improving the health of their populations, Sierra Leone focuses more on the objective of building a strong health system. Strengthening human resources for health, as well as disease and surveillance systems, are all key priorities. These priorities are in line with the lessons learned from the crisis in these countries, as well as with the advice provided by the international development community.

Assessment of National Investment Plans vis-à-vis Health Systems Strengthening and Universal Health Coverage

The widely recognized health systems strengthening framework proposed by the WHO was used to frame the analysis of the three post-Ebola national investment plans. The starting point of this framework was *The World Health Report 2000* on health system performance, which identified three generic goals and four generic functions of all health systems. The aim of any health system is to maximize the attainment of these goals, adjusted for the relative importance that a country attaches to each and conditioned by contextual factors from outside the health system that influence the level of goal attainment that can be reached (for example, a country's income, education levels, political factors, and so on). A simplified depiction of this framework is shown in figure 2.1.

The WHO subsequently reconfigured these four functions into six essential and mutually reinforcing "building blocks" of health systems, namely: (1) service delivery; (2) health workforce; (3) information; (4) medical products, vaccines, and technologies; (5) financing; and (6) governance (stewardship). These building blocks are geared toward helping countries achieve universal health coverage (UHC), which is defined as *"a system-wide effective health service coverage combined with universal financial protection."* In a strong health system, these building blocks interact in a manner that enables all people to access health care services when they need them without being impoverished by the costs of such services.

FIGURE 2.1
Health System Functions and Goals

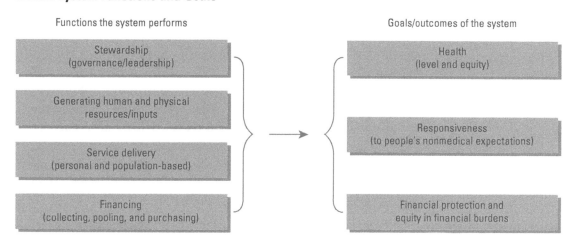

Source: Adapted from Duran et al., 2011.

FIGURE 2.2
The Dimensions of Universal Health Coverage: The UHC Cube

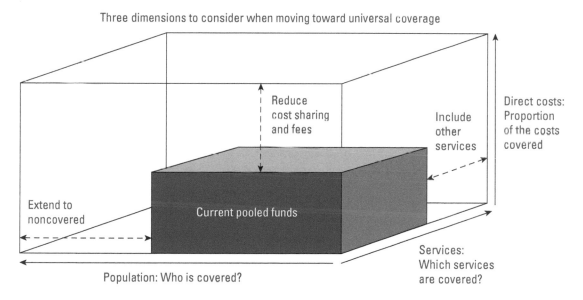

Source: WHO 2010.

The World Health Report 2010 depicted three *dimensions* of coverage as the axes of a cube: population, services, and costs (figure 2.2). The population axis describes the UHC objective of population coverage with both services and financial protection. The costs coverage axis is critical to the financial protection objective, although it needs to be interpreted relative to capacity to pay. And by defining the services coverage axis in terms of needed and effective services, this dimension captures the objectives of ensuring that everyone is able to use the health services that they need and that these services are of good quality. These three dimensions connect closely to health financing policies related to UHC and to the monitoring of UHC.

The path to UHC is thus one of strengthening the six health systems building blocks, and to make important policy decisions on the appropriate organization, the use and allocation of pooled funds that influence the direction and progress of reforms toward universal coverage (that is, to extend coverage to individuals previously not covered, to extend coverage to services previously not covered, and to reduce the direct payment needed for services).

Although the scope and reach of the investment plans in the three countries vary as a result of the different needs, contexts, and available resources, all the plans include relevant initiatives to strengthen the six essential building blocks of effective health systems proposed by the WHO in 2007. The baseline, moderate, and aggressive costing scenarios proposed by each country represent a recognition of the fact that the extent to which the health systems in each country can be strengthened is contingent on the quantum of resources that might be available. The pragmatic choice made by all three countries to pursue the baseline scenario, which represents the most basic level of systems development required to sustain the health sector, reflects the fact that the resources for health systems strengthening from both domestic and international sources are likely to be limited in the current global financial environment. Viewed in terms of health spending per capita, the costs associated with the proposed health plans are reasonable, even when compared with average health expenditures in Sub-Saharan Africa.

The strategic plans express the national vision, but more progress is needed on their translation into operational plans in order to realize that vision. In Liberia, using the investment plan as a blueprint for rebuilding and reinforcing the health sector, the Ministry of Health, together with development partners, has been engaged both in the development of detailed plans and guidelines for individual pillars and for their associated priority topics, and in establishing associated implementation arrangements. The latter include thematic working groups for coordinated planning, implementing, and tracking the progress of key pillars of the investment plan. In Guinea, a medium-term expenditure framework has been prepared. Its estimated costs are 19.7 percent higher than those of the investment plan for the period 2016–18. In Sierra Leone, there has been a similar consultative process to translate the plans into operation plans, and the government has taken some key steps to facilitate their implementation, such as a restructuring of the National Pharmaceuticals Procurement Unit to improve drug availability and reduce total costs. However, this process needs to be followed through to its logical conclusion.

The next section presents each building block in turn, and examines the salient features of the investment plans from the three countries vis-à-vis the definition of each building block provided in the WHO framework.[1] Suggestions are also made on how the investment plans might be improved, based on global best practices and experience.

Building Block 1. Service Delivery: Good health services are those that deliver effective, safe, quality personal and nonpersonal health interventions to those who need them, when and where needed, with a minimum waste of resources.

Status: The collapse of even routine health services as a result of Ebola is the single most important and immediate concern in the three countries. Specific issues that the countries face in the area of service delivery include (1) a breakdown of the critical elements for the delivery of a basic package of health services (for maternal and child health, communicable disease control, and key NCDs), including both facility-based and population-based services; (2) the lack of an effective referral system; (3) challenges in ensuring patient and health care worker safety, including infection prevention in health care units; (4) severe gaps in diagnostic and imaging service capacities; and (5) the limited participation of communities in the delivery of health services.

Issues addressed in plans: All three countries identify infection prevention and control, triage, and diagnostic capacity as key areas, and include specific interventions to address these issues. These interventions contribute to safe and effective health services, as well as to quality assurance, which have been highlighted by Guinea and Liberia. Part of effective care is the efficiency of the intervention; Guinea and Sierra Leone focus on high-impact interventions in maternal and child health, vaccination, and malaria control. They also focus on HIV/AIDS and tuberculosis (TB) control; in 2014, the incidence of TB per 100,000 population was 177 in Guinea, 308 in Liberia, and 310 in Sierra Leone.[2] Effective care is also fostered by facilities that have the necessary equipment and infrastructure, which Liberia and Sierra Leone identify as a priority. Guinea's investment plan notes the importance of traditional medicine for less-fortunate households and therefore seeks to integrate traditional providers into the health system; Liberia also seeks to regulate this sector and link it to the formal sector. Another aspect of effective health services is referral, which is included in Sierra Leone's plan. Of all the countries,

Liberia is the only one to focus on the client experience, which aims to promote partnership in health service delivery.

Service Delivery: What Else Could Be Done?

There is a proliferation of vertical programs (often supported by donors) in the three countries at the expense of an integrated delivery of health care services, which can result in a lopsided distribution of resources and skewed access to care. Global evidence suggests that, while effective and sometimes necessary in the short term, vertical programs can undermine the longer-term sustainability of health services. As countries move along the continuum from relief to development to economic growth and greater prosperity, greater integration of health systems is likely to lead to greater health gains.

As part of implementation, the countries should also consider a greater involvement of the private sector (both nonprofit and for-profit) in the delivery of services. Although government-financed, government-provided health services may be necessary in some situations (for example, for public and merit goods, targeting the poor, and so on), the private sector is a positive, powerful, and often underutilized force in health care delivery. Global evidence suggests that the private sector, if regulated effectively, is capable of providing high-quality care to large segments of the population—often more cost-effectively than government-run health services.

The countries should also place greater emphasis on leveraging modern technology in medical diagnostics and therapeutics, since this can often offer an effective substitute for scarce health human resources and can also prove to be cost-effective.

For health service delivery to be more effective and sustainable, specific steps must be taken to engage communities, so that providers, payers, politicians, and managers alike are held accountable, and the beneficiaries feel a sense of ownership of the services provided. This has been alluded to in the investment plans, but global evidence suggests that realizing the objective of community participation and ownership requires a high level of government commitment, targeted interventions, and significant capacity building.

Finally, the role of "implementation science" in gathering evidence on the relative costs and effectiveness of various service delivery approaches cannot be overemphasized. Linking any proposed intervention to proper monitoring and evaluation is critical. Although this is referred to in the plans, more emphasis and resources to support such evidence gathering and use are therefore warranted.

Building Block 2. Health Workforce: A well-performing health workforce is one that works in ways that are responsive, fair, and efficient to achieve the best health outcomes possible, given available resources and circumstances (that is, there are sufficient staff, fairly distributed; and they are competent, responsive, and productive).

Status: The EVD crisis has exposed the vulnerabilities of health systems that have dire shortages of health workers and significant labor market failures. The preexisting health workforce issues of extremely low numbers and densities—in particular, the highly uneven distribution of the workforce, which results in a higher density of workers in urban areas than in rural ones—were already common prior to the epidemic and have been further exacerbated by the EVD crisis across the three countries (see chapter 3 for details). This was exacerbated by weak competencies (including disease surveillance and response) and suboptimal health worker performance, particularly affecting health workers in the more remote parts of each country.

Issues addressed in plans: All three countries recognize the importance of strengthening human resources for health in terms of scaling up overall numbers and improving their distribution and performance. The investment plans of Guinea, Liberia, and Sierra Leone propose scaling up the overall production of health workers, with the former two aiming to reach a set of defined-density targets. All three countries put forward education- and incentive-related strategies that seek to improve the distribution and performance of health workers. Chapter 3 assesses the plans on human resources for health in greater detail (with each of the proposed interventions summarized in detail in appendix B.1), in particular the implications of reaching the proposed targets on cost, production capacity, fiscal absorption capacity, and distribution.

Health Workforce: What Else Could Be Done?

Chapter 3 provides detailed suggestions that can be discussed with the three countries vis-á-vis next steps. A central message is that in order to achieve the aim of a "fit-for-purpose" health workforce, particular attention should be directed toward *who*, *how*, and *where* health workers are trained and educated. Public sector funding should be directed particularly toward education and health workforce strategies with the largest social returns of investment, while the private sector could focus on education with large private returns on investment.

Global evidence suggests that a focus on preservice education programs that are outcome oriented and adopt innovative strategies for producing a fit-for-purpose workforce and skill mix that is appropriate to meet needs for UHC (particularly in remote areas) can be a powerful strategy to achieve medium- to longer-term results. Together with evidence-based financial and nonfinancial incentive programs, such strategies could improve the overall skill mix and distribution, as well as the performance, of health workers in the three countries, and ensure greater future resilience. Training, supervision, mentoring, and the use of a variety of quality assurance and quality improvement methods can garner shorter-term results and have equally been shown to be effective in raising standards of care. These need to be emphasized in the course of the implementation of the investment plans.

What is critical, overall, is that the design of specific interventions is based on a health labor market assessment of each country, to identify the demand- and supply-side dynamics of the health labor market so that appropriate constraints and solutions can be identified. Furthermore, more evidence should be generated on the relative costs and effectiveness of various approaches. Linking any proposed health worker interventions to impact evaluations is thus critical.

Building Block 3. Health Information Systems: Well-functioning health information systems are those that ensure the production, analysis, dissemination, and use of reliable and timely information on health determinants, health system performance, and health status.

Status: All three countries have weak routine health monitoring and evaluation systems, resulting in an undue reliance on population surveys. The data generated through the existing routine monitoring and evaluation systems are often ad-hoc and pro-forma, not collected in a timely manner, rarely vetted, and often paper-based. Collation and analysis capacity is limited, and the culture of analysis of data and its use for decision making at any level is virtually nonexistent. Even where data are collected (as in the case of certain vertical programs), the private sector is not included, which results in huge gaps in the data and compromises policy making. Evaluation is even more poorly developed than the monitoring of health care programs and interventions, and health research that might guide policy is almost never undertaken. Finally, the systems for integrated disease surveillance and response are rudimentary at best in the three countries, do not focus adequately on animal health (in line with the OneHealth principles), and very little attention is given to cross-border collaboration for disease surveillance and response.

Issues addressed in plans: All three countries focus on improving their health information systems. Disease surveillance systems, which are examined in detail in chapter 4, are part of the response in all three countries, although Liberia is the only country to provide a discussion of its planned implementation of the International Health Regulations

(IHR 2005) for disease surveillance. The approaches vary across countries, with Guinea focusing on coordinating Health Management Information Systems (HMIS) components and improving data quality with norms and audits; Liberia focusing on strengthening and harmonizing a set of systems;[3] and Sierra Leone seeking to strengthen its health information system. Guinea also points to various avenues for the production of health information beyond disease surveillance, such as annual National Health Accounts (as does Liberia) and strengthened medical research.

Health Information Systems: What Else Could Be Done?

Additional support is necessary to realize the three countries' aspirations regarding strengthening HMIS and other routine information systems. Indicators and their sources vary across the investment plans. As *The Roadmap for Health Measurement and Accountability* (World Bank Group, USAID, and WHO 2015) highlights, "Routine facility health information systems should be transparent, apply data management standards and include data quality assurance processes and verification through periodic samples of health services assessments." One way to test the commitment to HMIS strengthening is to determine the number of rows in the monitoring matrices that rely on facility survey data. Guinea has 15 percent (10/66), Liberia has none, and Sierra Leone's plan does not have a monitoring matrix, although the final review of its 2010–15 National Health System Strengthening Plan relies heavily on survey data and makes note of severe challenges for the HMIS.[4] Annual facility surveys, which are costly, do not directly strengthen the HMIS and cannot replace supervision functions that are also weak.

Civil registration and vital statistics should be part of well-functioning health information systems, and implementation support is therefore necessary in the recording of both births and deaths (including causes). Although the functionality of these systems varies across the countries, with all three countries self-evaluating them as being relatively weak and/or uncoordinated, Sierra Leone is the only country to explicitly plan for reinforcing this system in its health system strengthening plan. Sierra Leone will start by developing a national strategic plan and will include the use of the ICD-10 manual for recording causes of death. Liberia also has plans for strengthening its civil registration and vital statistics system, although specific proposals are not written into the country's national health plan. These efforts would very much benefit from best practice examples from other developing countries that have embarked on such programs.

Strengthening planning capacity is envisaged in all plans, with a focus on linking budgets to results, but more needs to be done. In the context of strengthened HMIS and other monitoring systems, such capacity building should strengthen the efficiency of resource allocation and use and may help to address equity challenges. However, only Guinea and Liberia provide detailed discussions of how to strengthen the capacity of their ministries of health, while Sierra Leone focuses more on donor coordination.

The management of health information using available electronic tools and information technology is essential as an enabler of access to quality and affordable health services. All three countries still primarily use paper-based systems to manage supply chains, clinical information, and monitoring and reporting. However, experience shows that the adoption of electronic record systems does not generate immediate, short-term results; therefore, rather than aiming at the ideal or optimum, modular, incremental approaches to digitization of health data can achieve early results and establish the foundations for future, more complex, interventions. In addition, investments in modern information technology and leveraging the capacity and reach of cell phone and Internet service providers can provide innovative and very efficient ways to collect, process, and disseminate the information that is required to improve health systems performance.

Building Block 4. Medical Products, Vaccines, and Health Technologies: Well-functioning health systems ensure equitable access to essential medical products, vaccines, and technologies of assured quality, safety, efficacy, and cost-effectiveness, and ensure their scientifically sound and cost-effective use.

Status: All the countries have poorly functioning pharmaceutical procurement and logistics systems, with a limited ability to manage the supply of essential medicines and supplies across the various levels of the health system. Access to drugs is an issue because of the limited ability of the public system to negotiate the prices of medicines, and because of the high prices of drugs in the private sector. The capacity of public health laboratories, including blood banks, is extremely limited, and they are often starved of resources—technical, human, and financial. The quality of drugs circulating in the local markets is suspect, and there have been reports of a proliferation of fake and counterfeit drugs in these countries. And the rational use of drugs is virtually nonexistent in the countries, leading to huge inefficiencies and also increasing the risks to the health of the population.

Issues addressed in plans: Proper storage and distribution of essential medicines are a priority in the investment plans of all three countries. The effectiveness and efficiency of supply chains requires considerable improvement in all three of them. Sierra Leone intends to move from a "push" to a "pull" system (which is based on scientific estimations of needs/demands, rather than arbitrary, norm-based supplies), with the implied improvements in logistics management, to reduce drug wastage. Part of that process will be to continue the process of developing its National Pharmaceuticals Procurement Unit. Liberia also plans to develop a logistics management information system to better manage drugs and reduce waste. Quality assurance and regulation, two essential elements, are a focus for Guinea and Liberia, which face high levels of illicitly imported and potentially substandard or counterfeit drugs. Guinea explicitly focuses on rational drug use, the scientifically sound and safe use of drugs, particularly through better treatment guidelines, the reduction of self-medication, and the proper dispensing of drugs.

Medical Products, Vaccines, and Health Technologies: What Else Could Be Done?

The plans for strengthening pharmaceutical logistics, pharmaceutical quality assurance, and the rational use of drugs are fairly comprehensive; however, operationalization of these plans will be the key to ensuring efficient and equitable pharmaceutical access and quality.

Regarding supply systems, several vertically funded family planning, vaccination, HIV/AIDS, TB, and malaria programs, with drug supply logistics systems built in, have been implemented in the three countries and have resulted in increases in commodity availability. This must continue, but with greater local participation in covering costs, in order to promote sustainability. In addition, the countries must be supported in leveraging their experience with the vertical pharmaceutical supply systems to build unified health sector supply chains that ensure the consistent availability of essential medicines at all service delivery points.

The effective implementation of a pricing policy has the potential to reduce the cost burden on the pharmaceutical system, reduce the prices of available medicines, and eliminate perverse incentives for pharmacies to push specific products that are more remunerative than others. The governments of the three countries will, however, need to actively engage the affected stakeholders in discussions and get their buy-in before finalizing pricing policies. On the financing side, in addition to government funding, a move toward public health insurance that includes reimbursement for medicines would reduce considerably out-of-pocket payments and promote access to good-quality medicines. Overall, a comprehensive pricing and patient access policy framework needs to be developed that can ensure effective, appropriate, equitable, and sustainable access in the context of UHC.

Finally, for effective pharmaceutical regulation and access to medicines, regional harmonization and cooperation are increasingly required. Pharmaceutical regulation is a complex process that aims to protect and promote public health. With increasing globalization, pharmaceutical production and distribution supply chains are getting more complex and challenge oversight by national regulatory bodies. There is an increasing global threat from pharmaceutical crime, and poor regulatory supervision of medicine production and distribution at all stages of the supply chain in all countries of the world generally, and in developing countries in particular. Regional initiatives might therefore be required to sustain access to essential drugs and to protect the quality of medicines in the three countries.

Building Block 5. Health Financing: A good health financing system raises adequate funds for health in ways that ensure that people can use needed services and are protected from financial catastrophes or impoverishment associated with having to pay for them. It provides incentives for providers and users to be efficient.

Status: The systems for generating, pooling, allocating, and managing the financing of health services are very weak in the three countries; this hinders equitable and efficient access to health care at all income levels, but particularly for the poor. The government's financial contributions to the health sector are limited (particularly in Guinea), and developmental assistance (which is sizable in the case of Liberia) sometimes substitutes for, rather than supplements, government financing. Out-of-pocket expenditures are therefore high, leaving the population economically vulnerable because of catastrophic and impoverishing health care costs. The limited fiscal space—coupled with inadequate institutional capacities, governance issues, and weak incentive systems—are major impediments to financial sustainability.

Issues addressed in plans: Health financing is particularly important because out-of-pocket expenditures are high in Guinea and Sierra Leone. At levels above 60 percent of total health expenditures, this means that populations are at risk of becoming impoverished by health care emergencies and that financing for the health systems is regressive. Another major source of financing is donors and NGOs, which present the risk of unpredictable resources, particularly as the postcrisis period advances. All three countries aspire to develop elements of social insurance or national health insurance schemes. These present the advantage of risk pooling and predictable expenditures, thus lowering the risk of impoverishing expenditures. Such risk pooling may be combined with financing from general revenues—as part of government health expenditures—to finance subsidized care for the poorest segments of the population, with a view to attaining universal coverage with essential health services. However, the investment plans neither provide sufficient detail nor allocate sufficient funding to implement such insurance programs within the context of a broad sectoral financing strategy.

Health Financing: What Else Could Be Done?

The investment plans from the three countries are, on the whole, weaker on health financing than in their treatment of the other health services strengthening building blocks. In order to address this gap, Guinea, Liberia, and Sierra Leone could learn from good practice examples of approaches to ensuring sustainable health sector financing in other developing countries. The pooling of health resources into insurance schemes and the development of innovative social protection mechanisms has been shown to be able to provide for universal coverage of a basic package of primary health services, particularly for the poorest members of society. There are many documented examples of countries where the progressive move toward UHC has been supported by strengthening the health financing systems. Two such examples, from Rwanda and Ghana, are provided here (see boxes 2.1 and 2.2). These country experiences can help guide Guinea, Liberia, and Sierra Leone in their efforts to develop

---

BOX 2.1

Rwanda: Combining Financial Protection and Results-Based Financing

With support from development partners, Rwanda engaged in a national scaling up of Community Based Health Insurance (CBHI) in early 2000. The enrollment rate had reached more than 90 percent in 2011. Because the CBHI beneficiaries are mainly poor or vulnerable and compose a large segment of the population, the government introduced a co-financed CBHI system, whereby other financial protection schemes covering formal sector workers make an annual share contribution (about 1 percent of their annual resources) to the CBHI. In addition, the government contributes to the CBHI fund to further boost pooling in an effort to cover the deficit. The poorest, who can prove they cannot afford the premiums (using the existing criteria for wealth ranking at the community level), have their premiums covered by the government, some development partners, and faith-based organizations. Concomitantly, performance-based financing was scaled up countrywide in Rwanda in 2006. With universal health coverage, and the use of a performance-based financing approach to improve health workers' motivation to deliver quality and health services, Rwanda has been acknowledged by the international community as a good example for other low- and middle-income countries to improve coverage and protect their populations from out-of-pocket expenditures, while also improving delivery of health services through the supply-side.

Source: WHO 2010.

BOX 2.2
Ghana: Health Insurance in Tandem with Decentralization

Since 2003, Ghana's National Health Insurance Scheme (NHIS) has been the main focus of efforts to reduce financial barriers to health services, complementing the Community-Based Health Planning and Services program that was launched in 1999 to reduce geographical barriers to health services access, particularly in remote rural communities. There has also been a complementary investment in the strengthening of district health systems with a view to improving health outcomes. The NHIS is funded mainly by employers' and employees' contributions, social security transfers, and a partially earmarked value-added tax. The NHIS had been operational for nearly a decade when it reached 50 percent of the targeted population. Surveys show that the NHIS is associated with a much higher rate of service use in relation to self-reported need, particularly for the poorest segment of the population.

Source: Adapted by authors from Blanchet, et al., *Ghana Medical Journal*, June 2012.

---

viable health financing systems, which are a crucial building block for realizing their aspirations to provide UHC to their citizens.

In addition to the introduction of public health insurance, other health financing options—such as mobilizing additional resources, including the reprioritization of the health sector in the budget; improving technical and allocative efficiency in the use of health sector resources; and strengthening the budgetary and financial management systems and capacities—are discussed in detail later in this chapter.

Building Block 6. Leadership and Governance: Leadership and governance involves ensuring that strategic policy frameworks exist and are combined with effective oversight, coalition building, regulation, attention to system design, and accountability.

Status: Policy frameworks exist for effective leadership and governance of the health sector in the three countries, but need to be strengthened and updated in order to be consistent with the evolving global and regional landscape. The coordination and leadership of the health sector across the central and local levels, as well as cross-sectoral collaboration, also need to be strengthened. Although devolution of sectoral governance has occurred to varying degrees in the three countries, the efforts have often not been resourced adequately, and progress has therefore not been optimal. Finally, community involvement in the governance of the sector has been limited at best across all three countries.

Issues addressed in plans: All three countries intend to strengthen coordination and leadership functions at the central and decentralized levels.

Devolution of responsibilities is important in all the plans, which also discuss the need to considerably strengthen district health management teams
(or their equivalents). All three countries also intend to increase cross-
sectoral collaboration, although Liberia appears to be the only country to
have built this into the preparation of its plan. Sierra Leone already had a
medium-term expenditure framework as part of its plan, and Guinea has
developed one since the plan was finalized. Liberia is the only country to
explicitly define the content for the strengthening of fiduciary and monitoring capacities. All countries recognize the importance of strengthening
the involvement of communities in governance. This ranges from developing guidelines for their involvement (Sierra Leone) to ensuring their participation in planning and monitoring (Guinea and Sierra Leone) to
increasing accountability (Liberia).

Leadership and Governance: What Else Could Be Done?

It would be worthwhile for each of the three countries to undertake a
comprehensive review of the legal and technical framework of the sector
in order to ensure the effective operation of both public and private
health services and the protection of patients' health and rights.
This includes ensuring that the standards of care, targets of care, and
targets for coverage are set, monitored, and maintained and that services
are cost-effective.

Global experience shows that decentralization of more effective
leadership, management, and governance capacity, in conjunction with
allocation of access and control over material and financial resources to
lower levels of health systems, fosters local ownership and improves the
responsiveness of those services to the populations served. Although all
three countries intend to move in this direction, implementation will be
key. For example, the preferential allocation of local treasury and international development resources toward the decentralization of service
provision and management decision making from national to district level
is essential in this process. Also needed are support for improved planning, budgeting, and management of integrated district-level primary
care services; the adaptation of these functions to local community needs;
and the development of effective targeting and incentive systems.

Intersectoral collaboration mechanisms will also need to be strengthened, particularly given that determinants outside the health sector are
at least as important to improving health and nutrition outcomes as
sectoral determinants.

Finally, global experience shows that the involvement of communities
in the delivery of health services in a meaningful way plays a significant

role in strengthening accountability and oversight of the health system and giving the users a greater say in systems, which often also largely finance themselves.

Plan Costs and Estimated Resources

Estimates of the plans' costs have been prepared using a number of different tools, as summarized in table 2.1. Liberia and Sierra Leone have three scenarios; Guinea has one. Where there are multiple scenarios, a baseline scenario outlines the absolute minimal level of investments necessary to provide a basic level of health services to the population; an aggressive scenario outlines the optimal level of investments that must be put in place in order to build a resilient health system and mitigate against the recurrence of such epidemics; and a moderate scenario balances resources and ambitions. Table 2.2 summarizes the scenarios and resources of each of the three countries.

There are important differences in the costing approaches adopted by the three countries. Guinea performed Marginal Bottlenecks Budgeting (MBB) prior to feeding the aggregates to OneHealth; Liberia used ingredient-based costing, which involves building up activities from their components and led to a very detailed set of costing tables. Sierra Leone, like Guinea, used the OneHealth tool, but also provided detailed information on how the estimates of the activities and their costs from the OneHealth tool were modified in order to fit the local context. The comparability of the estimates across countries is also affected by the varied categorization used in the different countries, which requires some harmonization.

TABLE 2.1
Country Post-Ebola Investment Plans

Country	Investment plan and period covered	Costing method
Guinea	System Recovery Plan, Health (2015–2017), Ministry of Health, Republic of Guinea	OneHealth Tool[a] subsequent to an MBB analysis
Liberia	Investment Plan for Building a Resilient Health System 2015–2021, Ministry of Health, Government of Liberia, 12 May 2015	Own ingredient-based costing methodology in Excel
Sierra Leone	Health Sector Recovery Plan (2015–2020), Ministry of Health and Sanitation, Sierra Leone	OneHealth Tool[a] with modifications based on local context

Note: MMB = Marginal Bottlenecks Budgeting.
a. The OneHealth Tool is "a software tool designed to inform national strategic health planning in low- and middle-income countries." See the WHO's website at http://www.who.int/choice/onehealthtool/en/.

TABLE 2.2
Summary of Scenarios and Financial Resources, by Country
U.S. dollars, millions

Scenario	2015	2016	2017	2018	2019	2020	2021	2022	2023	2024	Total
Guinea											
1. Baseline	621	720	673	657	674	819	795	858	922	989	7,728
4. Resources	539	568	478	415	383	371	368	368	369	372	4,230
5. Gap	82	152	196	243	292	448	427	490	552	617	3,498
Liberia											
1. Baseline	126	117	118	124	133	142	149	n.a.	n.a.	n.a.	910
2. Moderate	191	197	191	192	213	236	242	n.a.	n.a.	n.a.	1,461
3. Best case	209	213	205	206	233	254	265	n.a.	n.a.	n.a.	1,585
4. Resources	157	142	121	127	127	128	129	n.a.	n.a.	n.a.	931
5. Gap (moderate)[a]	−34	−54	−70	−65	−86	−108	−113	n.a.	n.a.	n.a.	−530
Sierra Leone											
1. Baseline	101	96	99	96	94	97	n.a.	n.a.	n.a.	n.a.	583
2. Moderate	105	116	140	150	154	142	n.a.	n.a.	n.a.	n.a.	806
3. Aggressive	121	136	156	158	162	150	n.a.	n.a.	n.a.	n.a.	883
4. Resources (MTEF)	58	89	114	n.a.	n.a.	n.a.	n.a.	n.a.	n.a.	n.a.	262
5. Gap (moderate)[b]	−47	−27	−26	n.a.	n.a.	n.a.	n.a.	n.a.	n.a.	n.a.	−99

Note: MTEF = Medium-Term Expenditure Framework; n.a. = not applicable.
a. Negative gap values mean that resources are larger than requirements.
b. Sierra Leone's Medium-Term Expenditure Framework covers 2015–17, so the gap is not comparable to that of Guinea or Liberia, which cover longer periods.

In Liberia, it is not clear that the formula-based equipment and management costing is accurate, although it is internally consistent.[5]

The available information from the investment plans and the national budgets suggests that the cost estimates, and associated gaps, are generally far larger than the current level of resources (figure 2.3). The strength of Sierra Leone's approach is that it is based on the country's Medium-Term Expenditure Framework (MTEF), which had a three-year time horizon. Guinea and Sierra Leone's horizons for health systems strengthening are longer, but they do not have the same macro foundation and may therefore prove to be unstable over time.

FIGURE 2.3
Resources and Gaps for the Moderate Scenarios, 2015–18

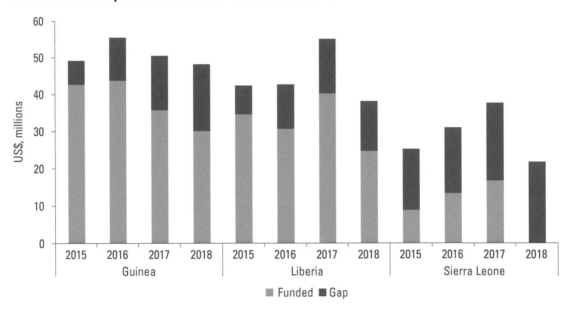

Sources: Guinea, Liberia, and Sierra Leone investment plans (2015–18).
Note: The data for Liberia is based upon fiscal 2015/16 to fiscal 2017/18.

Although the gap between what the investment plans estimate and what is available seem significant, especially for Guinea, it should be noted that the cost per capita of implementing the investment plans of the three countries remains reasonable, whether measured against the average per capita health spending in Sub-Saharan Africa (which has the least health spending among the world's regions) or the normative recommendations of the Abuja Declaration. For example, in Guinea, the recovery plan annual per capita cost does not exceed US$60 (versus an average of US$101 for Sub-Saharan African countries).

The three national investment plans do not have similar cost structures because the health systems in the three countries are different, and the conditions they were facing before the Ebola outbreak were also different. However, in all three cases, the cost projections are driven by the costs of infrastructure, equipment, drugs, surveillance, early detection, and response.

Unlike Liberia and Sierra Leone, Guinea does not show important human resource expenditure growth over time. After an initial expenditure of US$70 million in 2015, the Guinean investment plan's varying expenditures do not send a clear signal about human resource allocations.

Sierra Leone nearly doubles human resource allocations over time in the moderate and aggressive scenarios, and Liberia triples them for fiscal 2021/22 compared to the annualized fiscal 2014/15 level.

The scenarios suggest different constraints in Sierra Leone and Liberia. The largest constraints in Sierra Leone are service delivery and human resources; in Liberia they are infrastructure and epidemic preparedness. This is in part the result of the relatively higher, although absolutely low, level of human resources in Liberia as compared with Sierra Leone. These differing constraints have implications for the health systems strengthening process that are ongoing; in general, it may take less time—if the financial resources are forthcoming—to address the infrastructural issues compared to the human resource and service delivery constraints, which will require sustained attention and action. Chapter 3 analyzes the human resource picture in greater detail.

Health financing receives very uneven treatment in the investment plans of the three countries. Health financing is not mentioned in the Sierra Leone plan, despite the country's high dependence on out-of-pocket expenditures to finance its highly inequitable system. For Guinea, the main health financing objective is to define and implement a national health care financing strategy with a new scheme to cover the poorest. For Liberia, the objective is to put in place a sustainable health system that will ensure efficiency and equity in the use of health resources. Liberia goes further and aims to reinvigorate the process of establishing the Liberia Health Equity Fund, which aims to ensure sustainable financing for universal health coverage in the country.

For Guinea and Sierra Leone, it is important to ensure that the goal of achieving higher performance is not met at the expense of equity. In 2013, it was estimated that out-of-pocket spending financed 66 percent of health expenditures in Guinea and 76.2 percent of expenditures in Sierra Leone. This is unsustainable in the context of the massive additional financing requirement and already puts those with limited resources at risk of impoverishing expenditures, as discussed in the WHO's *The World Health Report* (2010). Universal health coverage elements of the plans will need to be carefully calibrated, given that the latest poverty estimates show that more than half the population in these countries is below the poverty line.

Governments will need to meet or exceed their domestic health financing commitments, even if donor resources reach desired levels. For Guinea, in particular, additional foreign resources have tended to displace domestic funds in the health sector. In an uncertain global macroeconomic environment, it is essential that domestic resources be executed as planned, and in an efficient manner, with joint monitoring by the countries and external partners to ensure that the international resources complement and do not substitute for domestic allocations. Available results for the 2015 and 2016 budgets are mixed; Sierra Leone executed 15.7 percent of its 2015 budget in favor of health (8.5 percent had been planned), and Guinea reached 4 percent in 2015, but was only able to increase it 15 percent more in 2016 rather than the planned doubling.

Previous experience suggests that supplemental resources often displace government financing. Table 2.3 shows regression coefficients for a model of government health expenditures as a linear function of external resources and private financing in the same time period over 1995/2013 based on the WHO National Health Accounts database. In all three countries, additional private resources lead to lower government financing, and in Guinea, additional external resources had the same effect. The "panel models" highlight that Guinea, Liberia, and Sierra Leone—as the "EVD countries"—behave differently than a larger West African pool of countries, which show less marked responses of government financing to other sources of funds.

Although it will undoubtedly be difficult to mobilize the resources required to finance the investment plans, ensuring the efficient execution of budgets that are far larger than the current levels may be the greater challenge. The government financial management and procurement systems in these countries are generally quite weak and will need to progress very rapidly in a human-resource constrained environment with massive

TABLE 2.3
Elasticity of Public Health Expenditures to Key Variables

Country	Contemporaneous						Average effect	
	Constant	External financing	Private financing	Adjusted R^2	F-statistic	Obser-vations	External	Private
Guinea	14.6***	−0.09**	−2.6***	0.96	206	19	−0.04	−3.0
Liberia	14.1***	−0.01	−2.5***	0.97	242	16		
Sierra Leone	19.2***	0.00	−3.7***	0.98	535	19	na	
	Panel models							
EVD countries	14.8***	−0.03***	−2.7***		1,228	54	Fixed effects	
Larger sample	9.0***	0.00	−1.3***		340	130	Random effects	

Source: WHO Global Health Expenditure Database, national health accounts, http://apps.who.int/nha/database.
Note: Averages are weighted by the number of observations. The larger sample includes the EVD countries and Côte d'Ivoire, Ghana, Nigeria, and Senegal. The Hausman test rejects the random effects specification for the EVD countries, but not for the larger set.
Significance level: ** = 5 percent, *** = 1 percent.

TABLE 2.4
Health, Population, and Reproductive Health Project Counts

Country	2007	2008	2009	2010	2011	2012	2013	2014
Guinea	145	142	209	162	208	194	214	257
Liberia	144	185	214	215	228	259	219	248
Sierra Leone	120	135	188	177	199	203	184	269

Source: OECD, Development Assistance Committee Creditor Reporting System.
Note: Sectors and subsectors in the Creditor Reporting System database are "I.2.a. Health, General," "I.2.b. Basic Health," and "I.3. Population Pol./Progr. & Reproductive Health."

injections of resources. Liberia, which enjoys the greatest donor resources, nearly quadrupled its executed budget over the fiscal 2007/08 to fiscal 2012/13 period, although the proportion of executed expenditures did not rise. In fact, in its fiscal 2013/14 budget, the execution rate fell even as the overall level also dropped.

Coordination and performance may require reducing the number of projects. According to the Creditor Reporting System of the Organisation for Economic Co-operation and Development (OECD), the three countries had more than 250 projects each in the health, population, and reproductive health sectors in 2014. Table 2.4 shows the numbers of projects per year. Of concern is that Guinea (50 percent in the period 2007–14), Liberia (62.5), and Sierra Leone (87.5) were at, or above, the median number of projects. Even if certain activities reflect donor-managed lines, all activities must still be coordinated. This is probably not feasible given the limited availability of personnel in the countries.

Fiscal Space

The next sections of this chapter assess and compare the fiscal space in each of the three countries since the Ebola epidemic, focusing on five dimensions: efficiency gains, external resources, macroeconomic environment, reprioritization, and sector-specific resources and taxation.[6] Pre-Ebola health financing levels and variability for the three countries are considered first; the current fiscal space situation, particularly in Guinea and Liberia, where the data are more detailed and allow such analysis, are then presented. Both the magnitude of possible revenues and their likelihood are taken into account, along with the relative importance of financing sources.

The pre-EVD health financing situation varied in the three countries most affected in important ways. For this analysis, data from the WHO

TABLE 2.5
Health Financing 2007–13: Levels and Variability

Average financing levels, 2007–13	Guinea		Liberia		Sierra Leone	
	Mean	**Standard deviation**	**Mean**	**Standard deviation**	**Mean**	**Standard deviation**
Health expenditures per capita (constant 2011 US$, purchasing power parity)	51.1	13.1	76.6	12.3	159.2	34.9
Out-of-pocket expenditures (% total)	57.6	10.0	30.5	4.9	68.7	7.4
External finance (% total)	21.1	8.5	52.2	8.5	30.6	12.8
Health in government budget (%)	6.6	2.5	14.5	3.0	11.6	1.1

Source: World Development Indicators from the World Health Organization's Global Health Expenditure Database, http://apps.who.int/nha/database. WHO data were updated on 23 May 2016.

are averaged for 2007 to 2013 to smooth fluctuations from individual years; the data include the first year of the EVD crisis (table 2.5). Sierra Leone had far higher total health expenditures per capita, but also the highest fluctuation in these levels. The country mobilized this high level of expenditures per capita primarily from households and external partners, despite its relatively high commitment to health (11.5 percent of the government budget). Across all three countries, external resources generally exhibit greater variation about their mean than do other sources of financing. The new WHO data extend the coverage to 2014. As might be expected, the total expenditures per capita rise with the addition of the first EVD year to the sample, but public health expenditures as a percentage of total government expenditures did not rise in Sierra Leone, and out-of-pocket expenditures rose in Liberia.

Macroeconomic Conditions

International Monetary Fund (IMF) revisions to GDP forecasts rule out growth as a source of fiscal space. Comparing the April 2016 and the October 2015 projections, GDP is revised down 5 percent in Guinea, 39 percent in Liberia, and 74 percent in Sierra Leone. Liberia had initially expected additional resources through revenue mobilization and the relatively large budget share of the sector (14 percent on average). Sierra Leone had expected to close 10 percent of the financing gap through this channel.[7] A recent editorial by the resident representative of the IMF in Sierra Leone cited statistics showing that the 60 percent decline in global iron ore prices in the 2014–15 period led to the closure of mines that represent 25 percent of Sierra Leone's economy and half of its exports. Furthermore, the editorial estimates that the combined effect of commodity prices and EVD contracted the economy by roughly 21.5 percent in 2015 and that the global commodities outlook for the medium term is not favorable (IMF 2015; Masha 2016).

Weak demand for raw materials could affect domestic financing in all three countries. Because the economies are resource dependent, a sustained weakness in the demand for raw materials could have important effects on the possibilities for domestic financing from growth, tax revenue, and out-of-pocket expenditures. For Guinea, mining is both a source of foreign direct investment and government revenue; the current decline in world primary commodity demand is a significant risk to its short- and medium-term macroeconomic outlook. Liberia's primary export commodities, iron ore and rubber, saw international prices decline by 50 percent and 35 percent, respectively, in 2014. For Sierra Leone, the primary sector is increasingly dominant (70 percent of GDP in 2014, up from 61 percent in 2012), and its composition is shifting toward mining and quarrying (20 percent in 2014, up from 3 percent in 2012), particularly iron ore (12 percent in 2014, up from 6 percent in the 2001–11 period).

The risk of a recurrence of Ebola exists, particularly if the health sectors are not rapidly strengthened. The first crisis was estimated by the World Bank to have cost US$2.2 billion in economic growth for 2015 alone.[8] A second shock might cost the three countries another 16 percent of GDP and would have major impacts on poverty and the overall macroeconomy beyond the ongoing commodity price shocks. Such a recurrence would reduce domestic resources for health further, and would likely make a future recovery more difficult. From an immediate demand-for-service perspective, various sources highlight the decline in reproductive and child health service demand, including immunizations, in the early Ebola period (Barden-O'Fallon et al. 2015; Bolkan et al. 2014; Menendez et al. 2015). This has immediate and longer-term consequences. Thus it may well make sense for the IMF to discuss with the three countries the possibility of relaxing the current ceilings for budgetary deficit financing (with necessary safeguards), to enable the countries to mobilize more resources for health, at least in the short run.

Reprioritization of the Health Sector in the Budget

All three countries have pledged to increase their health sector allocations. Guinea, which allocated only 1.9 percent of its 2012 budget to health, reached 4 percent in 2015, but only 4.6 percent in 2016, instead of the planned 6 percent. Financing for subsequent years is expected to be at least 6 percent. Liberia is already allocating between 8 and 12 percent of its budget to the health sector, so additional efforts may prove difficult without significant progress on health indicators (particularly the country's maternal mortality rate, which is 1,072 per 100,000 live births). Sierra Leone's MTEF figures indicate its ambition of doubling the total health budget (recurrent and capital costs) between 2015 and 2017. This will primarily come from 3.5 times more domestic capital resources; recurrent costs and transfers will increase by 25 percent in the same period.

Health efficiency must also rise to justify additional government resources. In the absence of additional borrowing, the budget formulation is a zero-sum process. A welfare-maximizing government must therefore choose among various options, making effective use of resources a higher priority. Choices related to level of care (primary, secondary, tertiary), type of care (curative or preventive), and location of facilities and staff (relative to populations) are extremely important. Beyond the discussion on human resources in chapter 3, examples of the type of care and level of care illustrate this. From its small health budget, Guinea allocated only 1.35 percent to five key health programs (vaccination, tuberculosis, malaria, HIV/AIDS, and Integrated Management of Childhood Illnesses); this is insufficient for Guinea's situation. In Liberia, two hospitals averaged 6.8 percent occupancy rates—at an average cost of US$278 per day—compared to less than US$200 per day in a random sample of other hospitals (World Bank Group et al. 2016).[9] This is in a country where total health expenditures per capita were US$42 per year over the 2009–13 period.

Earmarking Resources

Earmarking is not necessarily a stable solution. Taxation to finance a public good is a generally accepted principle, although issues of equity, transparency, simplicity, and universality must be considered. Under the assumption that these conditions are met, when it is legally feasible to allocate resources ex ante to specific sectors or activities, this may protect their budget allocation in the face of shocks. Earmarking, or the allocation of resources independently of the budget process, is not necessarily optimal because it reduces flexibility in allocation and may reduce overall allocative efficiency, although perhaps not at the levels considered in the three countries. Given that resources are fungible, an earmark may lead to a reduction of other sector resources if certain levels of resources are seen as normal; this produces an effective floor on resources, but may not increase them after the budgetary process runs its course. This effect may become stronger over time as the initial impetus for the earmark fades. Finally, earmarking resources without clear objectives and transparency in their use may not increase performance, particularly in weak governance environments where resources may be diverted to other uses.

Tax options are promising only in Guinea. Telephony-related taxes (currently dedicated to sectors affected by Ebola, including health), whether the taxes are on consumers or producers, could raise nearly US$67 million per year—an amount slightly larger than total government health spending in 2015. In Liberia, a package of allocations from the existing sin taxes (US$7 to US$13 million) and proposed motor vehicle insurance and registration fees (US$7 to US$14 million) could generate between US$14 million and US$27 million over a seven-year period. The baseline scenario gap would be reduced possibly by half if these resources were allocated directly to health. These options are not currently feasible in Sierra Leone, where the trend of rising tax exemptions and high tax avoidance rates (35 percent in 2015) may prove difficult to reverse, although the amounts of monies forgone through such exemptions and tax avoidance are equivalent to government health allocations in some years. The November 2015 IMF report also identifies these elements as essential changes to achieve increased revenue, which was the key fiscal challenge for 2016.

Mobilizing Additional Resources

The financing strategies of all three countries rely heavily on two resources: out-of-pocket expenses and donors. Out-of-pocket expenses are discussed later in this book. Pre-Ebola, Guinea mobilized roughly 10 percent of its health spending from donors—less than Liberia (35 percent) or Sierra Leone (15 percent). In the costing plans, donor resources represent 30–53 percent for Guinea (2015–18), 50–60 percent for Liberia (fiscal 2015/16 to fiscal 2021/22), and Sierra Leone (2017 and 2018). Although this finding suggests that Guinea and Sierra Leone might try to mobilize additional donor funds, the extent to which such external support might be forthcoming is an open question.

Supply-side risks: The important effort made by donors during the Ebola period may not be sustained in the medium term and represents a very large risk to the overall financing plan. Such levels of dependence introduce multiple risks: shocks to service delivery if donors reduce levels, the potential inability to finance recurrent costs (for example, in 2014/15, 39 percent of Liberia's recurrent health expenditures were covered by on-budget donor funds), and displacement of domestic resources away from health.

Demand-side risk: The three countries are at "moderate risk" of debt distress.[10] This status increases the importance of concessional funding, may limit domestic borrowing in light of tighter fiscal positions (Sierra Leone), rapidly increase public debt (Guinea), and introduce the risk of further negative commodity shocks (Liberia). Sierra Leone is particularly limited because the recent commodity shocks have brought it close to being at high risk of debt distress. What this implies is that governments will need to rely on concessional financing and to prioritize health over other possible sectors to support their plans while remaining within debt sustainability parameters. For example, Liberia's external financing ceiling for 2016 is set at US$180 million in nominal terms, which means that between 30 and 39 percent of its borrowing limit would need to be devoted to the national plan for the moderate and aggressive scenarios, respectively. The IMF report notes that this may require "significant streamlining of new concessional agreements compared to the pipeline."

All three EVD-affected countries have a significant share of private health spending relative to total spending, as shown in figure 2.4.

FIGURE 2.4
The Relative Importance of Health Financing Sources, 2012 and 2013, Selected Countries

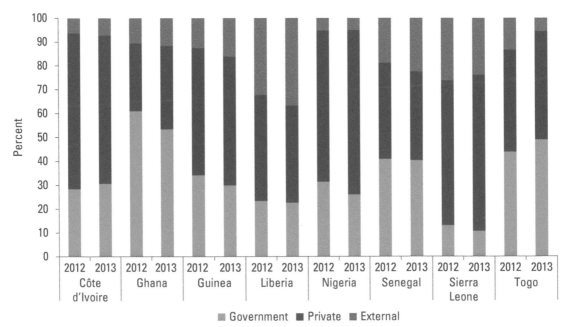

Source: The World Health Organization's Global Health Expenditure Database, http://apps.who.int/nha/database.
Note: Data are rescaled to sum to 100 percent as the underlying series do not do so.

This is particularly important in Sierra Leone, where government resources are quite limited. While the effects of the macro economy may not immediately translate to the household level, the effects of EVD seem to be less in doubt. Both the World Bank's work on the impact of the crisis in Liberia (Himelein and Kastelic 2015) and a recent preliminary report by the World Food Program (CFSVA 2016) suggest that livelihoods were significantly affected. In late 2015, food insecurity was rising, income was not higher than it had been in pre-EVD times, and livelihoods (particularly fishing) had been seriously affected. In turn, households may not be able to sustain the prior rates of funding.

Improving Efficiency

The potential to increase efficiency exists in all three countries. Increased efficiency may be studied through two lenses: allocative and technical efficiency. As the WHO's *World Health Report* (2010) suggests, all countries have some degree of inefficiency, which varies. Each country is considered in turn below.

Strengthening public financial management (PFM) is an essential part of increased efficiency. The latest IMF country reports and press releases all highlight the need to "strictly apply the PFM code include procurement for efficient use of public resources" (Guinea), to "address PFM" (Liberia), and to "deepen PFM reforms" (Sierra Leone).[11] Without these structural changes and performance enhancements, there is a high risk that additional resources will either not be executed (for example, by virtue of a slowdown in Liberia's execution of donor funds) or may not be optimally utilized, for various reasons.

Guinea's allocative efficiency is characterized by an inequitable allocation of human and financial resources and insufficient support for basic public health programs that have a large impact and positive spillovers. For example, in Conakry, only 4 percent of mothers do not have an antenatal care visit and 9 percent are not assisted by trained staff. This is clearly not the case for the rest of the country, which has far lower rates. Using a measure of needs that sums antenatal care, births assisted by trained staff, and child vaccination rates, Conakry has a need of 47, while the country as a whole scores 139. Since staff are concentrated in urban areas and their remuneration is the largest line item in the health budget, this creates the observed inequality that Conakry receives over half of the country's total health funding. This inequity in resource allocation is compounded by massive underspending on basic health programs—only 2.7 percent of resources goes toward 18 public health programs; 1.35 percent goes toward vaccination, tuberculosis, malaria, HIV/AIDS, and Integrated Management of Childhood Illnesses. Finally, resources allocated to the ministry appear to not be explicitly designated to a particular program, which suggests inefficiency and a lack of transparency (World Bank 2014).

In Liberia, the health system is inefficient, both in the allocative and in the technical sense. There are insufficient ancillary inputs available (when needed) at all levels of care to diagnose and treat the ailments presented. And given the low number of patients presented per facility per week, say, many government clinics are experiencing an oversupply of staff relative to the amount of work they do. There are some, of course, that are relatively understaffed for some reason. In the current instance, saving money by reducing staff (to make health services more efficient, in this case) is impossible. In fact, one may have to raise resource inputs first before efficiency gains could be considered as a source of new funding. From this perspective, gains from efficiency, in the realm of health services delivery, are generally very difficult to achieve, and certainly to maintain (World Bank Group et al. 2016). A similar situation is observed in Sierra Leone, where the 2014 report from the Office of the Auditor General showed that 90 percent of peripheral health units do not have essential equipment needed to provide quality service and that many hospitals are lacking basic obstetric equipment.

For Sierra Leone, one source of allocative efficiency that stands out is improving public financial management. Since there is no centralized accounting of revenues, the estimated US$214.5 million spent by patients in the public sector in 2013 was not recorded in the government's ledgers. Given the very low levels of support, this may simply mean that funds were used to pay for inputs, but clearly information to guide allocations was missing. However, the low funding levels have another consequence: illegal fees are added by facilities to compensate for initiatives such as the Free Health Care Initiative for children under the age of five and pregnant and lactating mothers (18.5 percent of total health expenditures in the 2013 National Health Accounts). According to the latest IMF supervision report (November 2015), the authorities had already begun publishing monthly reports on donor funds channeled through the National Ebola Response Center and intended to begin publishing quarterly reports on funds that are on budget.

Improving resource management may effectively be a source of increased revenues. The Sierra Leone fiscal space analysis estimates that unaccounted revenue will represent 9 percent of its domestic health budget in 2017. Resources collected by health facilities are not reported to the ministries of health or finance, and are therefore not included in programming. In this vein, Liberia plans to strengthen resource tracking and accountability.

Technical efficiency is harder to measure without explicit studies, but some evidence is suggestive. Guinea's maternal mortality ratio lies above the regression line for purchasing-power-parity income per capita for countries in the region, suggesting that it is not getting value for money. The fiscal space analysis report for Guinea estimates that the lack of progress on the health Millennium Development Goals resulted in 18,500 avoidable maternal and child deaths in 2012, which is equivalent to a loss of 4.8 percent of GDP. For Liberia, it appears that although lower-level facilities lack inputs needed to deliver services, tertiary care hospitals appear to be run in a highly inefficient manner, with very high costs per day and correspondingly low bed occupancy rates. This observation is corroborated by an internal comparison of lower-level hospital costs for patients, which are seven to twenty times cheaper than the costs for patients in tertiary care hospitals on average.[12] This may also spill over into equity, as there is a sixfold variation in per capita spending across counties in Liberia, ranging from US$6 (Grand Kru) to US$1 (Nimba), with most receiving roughly US$2 per capita.

Conclusions

The six essential building blocks for health systems strengthening, defined by the WHO (2007), serve to frame the discussion above and provide an approach to health systems strengthening in the three countries. The costed national investment plans prepared by the three governments are presented and compared, and the chapter analyzes their viability, realism, and implications in relation to the WHO health systems strengthening framework and the available health sector resources. Suggestions are then made on how the plans could be strengthened for each health systems building block.

The fiscal space analysis finds serious gaps between the resources required and the resources available for all three countries: governments will need to meet or exceed their domestic health financing requirements, even if donor resources reach desired levels. Furthermore, although it will undoubtedly be difficult to mobilize the resources required to finance the investment plans, ensuring the efficient execution of budgets that are far larger than the current levels may be the greater challenge. While all three countries have proposed an increase in their health budgets—and Guinea, in particular, has significantly increased its budgetary allocations (albeit from a low base)—the following considerations should guide the implementation of the plans:

- *Governance:* It is necessary for the three governments to define implementation strategies and processes that would optimize the achievement of health sector outcomes. The results of the analysis should be translated into multisectoral support for the health sector that explicitly links improvements in public financial management and sectoral decentralization to sector outcomes. At the World Bank, the program-for-results option may help to make this link explicit, particularly if resource allocation formulas are developed.

- *Planning:* Donors should reduce the number of projects financed through off-budget allocations in order to facilitate coordination and hence implementation. Technical assistance and human resource development will help to improve planning, particularly if decentralization of responsibilities in health increases. Plan monitoring should also be strengthened to motivate donors to avoid parallel systems, whether these systems are fiduciary or technical.

- *Strategies:* Financing strategies—both domestic and international—are needed to address the vulnerability stemming from a heavy reliance on out-of-pocket expenditures. These strategies should cover the macroeconomic, health, and social protection dimensions, given the levels of poverty and the countries' desire to move toward universal health coverage.

Recognizing the bleak macroeconomic prospects in the short to medium terms, the already high and inequitable levels of out-of-pocket health expenditures, and the limited scope for earmarked taxes to finance the health sector, recommendations for expanding the fiscal space for the investment plans in the three countries are to:

- *Improve donor coordination and ensure commitment:* Donors should move away from off-budget project financing toward pooled funds or, possibly, sector budget support in line with the Paris Declaration on Aid Effectiveness and the IHP+ principles.[13] It is essential that such pooling be linked to independently verifiable improvements in the performance of health systems, including measures of service delivery coverage and quality of care.

- *Improve allocative efficiency:* This may be done at the macro and subnational levels. First, sector Medium-Term Expenditure Frameworks (MTEFs) should be defined in coordination with macroeconomic MTEFs. In parallel, clear allocation rules for resources including staff should be defined.

- *Improve technical efficiency:* Among the primary areas of focus are fiduciary capacities, standards of care and regulation, supportive supervision, and alternative incentive schemes. The use of performance-based financing may help to increase fund flows, but will require increased supervision to ensure that the quality of care is not compromised. Ongoing performance-based financing efforts in Liberia and Sierra Leone may thus require adjustments, now that the immediate crisis of the Ebola outbreak has abated.

• *Improve data:* Insufficient and sometimes incoherent information hinders the efficient use of resources and may, in itself, create waste. National systems such as health and logistics management information require additional investments, as do donor coordination mechanisms. In general, strengthening information should avoid focusing excessively on surveys at the expense of routine systems and monitoring, in order to avoid perpetuating the existing problems.

The World Bank can play a pivotal role both in ensuring that sustainable progress is made in terms of health financing, and in advising the countries on options to increase the fiscal space for health. The World Bank has a comparative advantage and capacity in terms of technical assistance in the area of health financing, results-based financing, and evidence-based planning and budgeting. To increase fiscal space, the World Bank may be of assistance in three areas: (1) technical assistance in evidence-based planning and budgeting and the development of health financing and UHC strategies, (2) providing results-oriented lending, and (3) using its convening power to support the necessary changes.

Notes

1. Definitions for each of the six areas are from WHO (2007, vi).
2. See Global Health Observatory data repository, available at http://apps.who .int/gho/data/view.main.57040ALL?lang=en. In 2014, Guinea, Liberia, and Sierra Leone ranked 24, 15, and 16, respectively, in Sub-Saharan Africa.
3. These are a Health Management Information System, Logistics Management Information System, Financial Management Information System, integrated Human Resources Information System, and Community-Based System.
4. This is consistent with the conclusion of the first review of the Joint Program of Work and Funding in 2014, which found that a lack of monitoring of program implementation was a major weakness (5 percent was fully implemented, and 25 percent was partially implemented).
5. Administrative and management costs make up 5 percent of the implementation costs, and equipping new or enhanced infrastructure is estimated at 15 percent of the cost of constructing it, while maintaining it is estimated to cost 10 percent of its construction cost. This approach has the merit of considering these costs explicitly, but may not always provide accurate values.
6. This is based upon Heller (2005) and Tandon and Cashion (2010).
7. GDP growth increases the government health budget to US$70.4 million in 2018 (a 40 percent increase relative to 2016). This increase represents an additional US$3 per capita, but only 10 percent of the financing gap.
8. World Bank Economic Update on Ebola, April 17, 2015.

9. See the "Fiscal Space Analysis for Health in Liberia" (World Bank Group et al. 2016). Averages for the hospitals are weighted by total inpatient days.
10. This paragraph uses the conclusions of the latest IMF Country Reports for Guinea (16/95), Liberia (16/8), and Sierra Leone (15/323).
11. Ibid.
12. The comparison of costs for patients is somewhat difficult because lower-level hospitals lack basic inputs and tertiary hospitals may also deal with the most complex and challenging cases, but since it is based upon budgets rather than direct expenditures, all else being equal, it measures policy intent. The magnitudes are also large.
13. For information about the Paris Declaration on Aid Effectiveness, see http://www.oecd.org/dac/effectiveness/parisdeclarationandaccraagendaforaction.htm; for information about the International Health Partnership (IHP+) see http://www.internationalhealthpartnership.net/en/

References

Barden-O'Fallon, Janine, Mamadou Alimou Barry, Paul Brodish, and Jack Hazerjian. 2015. "Rapid Assessment of Ebola-Related Implications for Reproductive, Maternal, Newborn and Child Health Service Delivery and Utilization in Guinea." *PLOS Currents Outbreaks*, August 4. Edition 1. doi: 10.1371/currents.outbreaks.0b0ba06009dd091bc39ddb3c6d7b0826.

Blanchet, N. J., G. Fink, I Osei-Akoto. 2012. "The Effect of Ghana's National Health Insurance Scheme on Health Care Utilization." *Ghana Medical Journal* 46 (2): 76–84.

Bolkan, Håkon, Donald Alpha Bash-Taqi, Mohammed Samai, Martin Gerdin, and Johan von Schreeb. 2014. "Ebola and Indirect Effects on Health Service Function in Sierra Leone." *PLOS Currents Outbreaks*. December 19. Edition 1. doi: 10.1371/currents.outbreaks.0307d588df619f9c9447f8ead5b72b2d.

CFSVA (Comprehensive Food Security & Vulnerability Analysis). 2016. Preliminary Findings, WFP Sierra Leone Country Office. 10 February 2016.

Duran, A., J. Kutzin, J. M. Martin-Moreno, and P. Travis. 2011. "Understanding Health Systems: Scope, Functions, and Objectives." In *Health Systems, Health, Wealth and Societal Well-Being: Assessing the Case for Investing in Health Systems*, edited by J. Figueras and McKee, 19–26. Berkshire: Open University Press.

Himelein, Kristen, and Jonathan G. Kastelic. 2015. "The Socio-Economic Impacts of Ebola in Liberia: Results from a High Frequency Cell Phone Survey, Round 5." World Bank, Washington, DC. https://openknowledge.worldbank.org/handle/10986/21893.

IMF (International Monetary Fund). 2015. "Sierra Leone: Third and Fourth Reviews under the Extended Credit Facility Arrangement and Financing Assurances Review, Requests for Waivers for Nonobservance of

Performance Criteria and Modification of Performance Criteria, and Requests for Re-Phasing and Augmentation of Access under the Extended Credit Facility." IMF Country Report 15/323. IMF, Washington, DC.

———. 2016. "Fourth Review under the Extended Credit Facility Arrangement and Requests for Waivers of Nonobservance of Performance Criteria, Modification of Performance Criteria, and Re-Phasing and Extension of the Arrangement." IMF Country Report 16/8.IMF, Washington, DC.

Masha, Iyabo. 2016. "Sierra Leone's Economy in the Post-Ebola Era." An Op-Ed first published in Awoko Newspaper, reprinted on the IMF website. http://www.imf.org/external/np/vc/2016/011816.htm.

Menéndez, Clara, Anna Lucas, Khátia Munguambe, and Ana Langer. 2015. "Ebola Crisis: The Unequal Impact on Women and Children's Health." *The Lancet* 3 (3): e130. doi: http://dx.doi.org/10.1016/S2214-109X (15)70009-4.

World Bank. 2014. "Guinee: Revue des depenses publiques (PER). Public Expenditure Review (PER)." Washington, DC: World Bank Group. https://hubs.worldbank.org/docs/imagebank/pages/docprofile.aspx?nodeid=23138586.

World Bank, Ministry of Health of Liberia, WHO (World Health Organization), and Clinton Health Access Initiative. 2016. *Fiscal Space Analysis for Health in Liberia.* Final Draft. March 2016.

World Bank, USAID (U.S. Agency for International Development), and WHO (World Health Organization). 2015. *The Roadmap for Health Measurement and Accountability.* MA4Health, June. http://www.healthdatacollaborative.org/fileadmin/uploads/hdc/Documents/the-roadmap-for-health-measurement-and-accountability.pdf.

WHO (World Health Organization). 2000. *The World Health Report 2000: Health Systems: Improving Performance.* Geneva: WHO.

———. 2007. *Everybody's Business: Strengthening Health Systems to Improve Health Outcomes.* Geneva: World Health Organization.

———. 2010. *The World Health Report: Health Systems Financing—The Path to Universal Coverage.* Geneva: World Health Organization.

CHAPTER 3

Plans to Scale Up and Improve the Distribution of the Health Workforce

Introduction

The Ebola virus disease (EVD) outbreak crisis has exposed the vulnerabilities of health systems that have dire shortages of health workers and significant labor market failures. Preexisting health workforce issues of extremely low numbers and densities—in particular, the highly uneven distribution of the workforce, which results in a higher density of workers in urban areas—were already common prior to the epidemic and have been further exacerbated by the EVD crisis across the three countries.

Perhaps not surprisingly, the aim of strengthening the health workforce is a core feature of the post-Ebola investment plans of each country. Among other things, these plans seek to expand the availability of health workers at all levels of the health system, to cope with the breadth of the disease burden, and to be better prepared for future pandemics. Table B.1.1 (in appendix B.1) provides an overview of some of the health workforce areas on which each of the plans is focusing. The costing of the investment plans, discussed in the previous chapter, took into account the inputs needed to achieve certain targets for scaling up the health workforce.

Targets for health workforce scaling up can be derived both from the investment plans themselves and from the costing exercise that accompanies them, with notable differences. For all three countries, numerical targets for health workforce scaling-up plans can be derived from the detailed costing exercise of the investment plans. Only Guinea and Liberia included health worker density targets in their investment plans—targets that are to be achieved by 2021 and 2024, respectively, for certain cadres of health workers.

The objective of this chapter is to better understand the nature and implications of the proposed health worker scaling-up plans of the three countries, as specified in their investment plans and associated costing. It is not intended to be prescriptive, given that the investment plans and costing tools were developed through extensive consultations and by the political economy inherent to each country. Instead, the chapter dissects the scaling-up targets for human resources for health (HRH) for each of the countries and discusses the implications of reaching those targets, as well as international density thresholds, with regard to meeting the needs, graduate production output, and actual cost as well as the projected fiscal space available for HRH. In addition, the chapter discusses the implications of inaction to address rural/urban imbalances, and the extent to which existing country scaling-up plans may affect this imbalance. The conclusions and recommendations at the end of the chapter will be of use to all those aiming to understand and invest toward the HRH-related goals outlined in the investment plans.

Data

Health workers in this analysis are defined as all cadres employed in the service of health. This includes care providers (such as doctors, nurses, and midwives) as well as allied health professionals and administrative and support staff. The central analysis of this report, however, focuses on doctors, nurses, and midwives because of the existing evidence base around densities of such cadres and health service delivery outcomes. Data were coded into the major categories of cadres defined by the International Standard Classification of Occupations (ISCO-88). Health worker densities were derived by using 2015 population estimates.

Public sector payroll data from 2015 were used as the basis for the health workforce analysis. Payroll data are generally reflective of the public health workforce on government payroll; this is comparable across the three countries and likely represents the majority of the workforce in the country. Payroll data from 2015 do not reflect the results of recent payroll audits that have been completed in Liberia and Sierra Leone, in part to weed out "ghost workers" (those workers listed on the payroll but who are not actually working in the system). Payroll data, moreover, do not include health workers in the private sector (largely concentrated in the capitals in all three countries) although dual practices are likely to be common.

Payroll data in Guinea and Sierra Leone exclude some formal and informal health workers serving in the public sector. According to the

2014 census data, for example, 4,566 health workers who are in the public sector in Guinea are paid by nongovernmental organizations (NGOs) or provide services voluntarily. In Sierra Leone approximately 9,500 health workers providing services in the public sector are not on the payroll. In addition, health workers who are not formally contracted or part of the payroll but who provide services in the public sector are also prevalent; these workers range from an estimated 39 percent in Guinea (not included in the payroll list) to 48 percent in Sierra Leone (not included in the payroll list) and 44 percent in Liberia (included in the payroll dataset but not paid by the government). This should be taken into account as the analysis presented in this chapter reflects workforce density as per the payroll data.

Health worker information systems across all three countries require investments to strengthen their reliability and comprehensiveness because they are often fragmented across multiple sources. Data required for a complete labor market analysis, taking into account current and future population needs, were incomplete or missing at the time of this analysis. This necessitated crude assumptions and scenarios regarding health worker training, costs of training, attrition, and distribution. Because of the lack of defined and cross-country comparability of rural and urban areas, with the exception of Guinea, the region including the capital city was crudely defined as urban and all other areas were defined as rural. The analysis and figures should thus be interpreted with these limitations in mind.

Health Workforce Stock and Distribution: The Current Public Sector Situation

This section provides a brief overview of the current stock, density, and distribution of (public sector) health workers in Guinea, Liberia, and Sierra Leone. Drawing on extensive analyses of 2015 government payroll data for each country, the analysis shows that the stock of health workers in all three countries is extremely low, although Liberia fares comparatively better on this front than Sierra Leone or Guinea (figure 3.1).

Liberia is ahead of both Guinea and Sierra Leone in terms of the availability of public sector workers, both in total numbers and in numbers of doctors, nurses, and midwives only. Although Guinea has the smallest stock of combined health workers (when all health worker categories are included), it has a very large stock of community health volunteers and the largest stock of doctors of the three countries. Liberia has the largest stock of mid-level cadres, and Sierra Leone has the largest stock of low-level cadres.

FIGURE 3.1
Number of Public Sector Health Workers, 2015

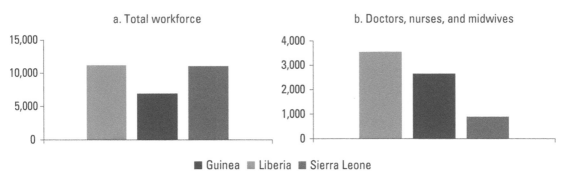

a. Total workforce   b. Doctors, nurses, and midwives

■ Guinea ■ Liberia ■ Sierra Leone

Source: 2015 government payrolls (public sector only).
Note: Total workforce includes all categories of staff employed in the public sector. *Doctors, nurses, and midwives* includes general medical practitioners, specialist medical practitioners, physician assistants, registered nurses and nurse professionals, and registered midwives and midwifery professionals (for example, certified midwives), and excludes nursing associate professionals such as nursing aides and assistants.

FIGURE 3.2
Health Worker Density, 2015

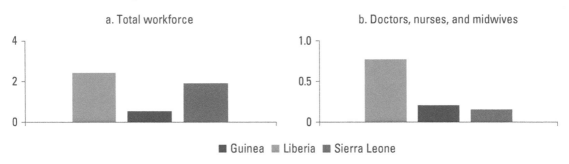

a. Total workforce   b. Doctors, nurses, and midwives

■ Guinea ■ Liberia ■ Sierra Leone

Source: 2015 government payroll and 2015 population data (CIA database).
Note: Total workforce includes all categories of staff employed in the public sector. *Doctors, nurses, and midwives* includes general medical practitioners, specialist medical practitioners, physician assistants, registered nurses and nurse professionals, and registered midwives and midwifery professionals (for example, certified midwives), and excludes nursing associate professionals such as nursing aides and assistants. DNM = doctors, nurses, and midwives.

Taking into account population levels, the ratio of health workers to the population (that is, the health worker density) is extremely low in all three countries, although density levels in Liberia are higher than they are in the other two. Liberia's higher health worker density in part may reflect its comparatively lower population levels: 4.6 million, compared to 5.7 million in Sierra Leone and 12.7 million in Guinea (figure 3.2).

The extremely low level of health workers in all three countries is highlighted when compared with regional averages (table 3.1). Current densities of doctors, nurses, and midwives in all three countries are far

TABLE 3.1
Average Densities of Doctors, Nurses, and Midwives, by Region, 2013

WHO region	Doctors	Nurses and midwives	Total
Africa	0.24	1.09	1.33
Americas	2.29	5.49	7.78
Eastern Mediterranean	1.01	1.42	2.43
Europe	3.25	6.81	10.06
South Asia	0.58	1.24	1.81
East Asia	1.87	2.51	4.37
Western Pacific	1.40	2.08	3.48
Global	1.36	2.75	4.11

Source: Global Health Observatory, World Health Organization (http://apps.who.int /ghodata/#).
Note: Density is defined here as the number per 1,000 population.

below the average of all regions, including Africa. Countries in Africa have an average doctor, nurse, and midwife density of 1.33 per 1,000 population, already far below the average of all other regions. Liberia, which has the largest density of all three countries, is close to half the African average (with 0.77), with Guinea and Sierra Leone falling even further behind (with 0.20 and 0.15, respectively).

The distribution of health workers is uneven in all three countries, although Liberia's workforce is more evenly distributed than the others, with 57 percent of doctors in rural areas and 43 percent in urban areas (the population distribution is 68 percent rural and 32 percent urban). In contrast, in Guinea 98 percent of doctors and 88 percent of nurses reside in urban areas, where only 36 percent of the population live; and in Sierra Leone, 92 percent of doctors and 72 percent of nurses reside in urban areas, where only 18 percent of the population live (figure 3.3).

Taking into account population densities, workforce distribution, while suboptimal in Liberia, is better than it is in Guinea or Sierra Leone. Liberia's health workforce is already more equally distributed across regions (and their populations) than that of Guinea and Sierra Leone. Figure 3.4 is a concentration index calculated from district-level workforce density for each country. If the distribution of the health workforce was proportional to the population size of each district, the curve would fall along the dashed line—the populations and workforce of each district are added cumulatively, so the accumulation of the population and the

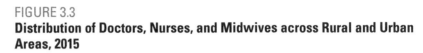

FIGURE 3.3
Distribution of Doctors, Nurses, and Midwives across Rural and Urban Areas, 2015

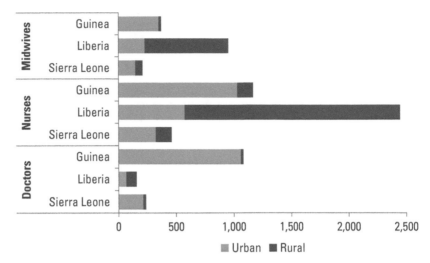

■ Urban ■ Rural

Note: Guinea's internal classification system of urban and rural was applied. Comparable rural and urban classifications were not available for Liberia and Sierra Leone, and thus the county or district with the capital was defined as the urban area with the remaining counties and districts classified as rural. In Liberia, the urban area was defined as Montserrado County; in Sierra Leone, the urban area was defined as the Western Area.

health workforce would occur at the same rate. In the figure, the curves for the Guinea, Liberia, and Sierra Leone health workforces all fall below the dashed line, indicating that the workforce is unequally distributed in all of them. For example, 40 percent ($x = 40$) of the total population who live in regions with lower health worker densities have approximately 20 percent of the health workforce in Sierra Leone, 22 percent of the health workforce in Guinea, and 30 percent of the health workforce in Liberia.

Health Worker Scaling-Up Ambitions and Implications by Investment Plans

This section discusses the nature and implications of the scaling-up plans of the three countries by assessing the targets for doctors, nurses, and midwives extracted from investment plan targets for scaling up. In line with the timeframe of the investment plans, health worker scaling-up plans in Guinea and Sierra Leone run until 2024 and 2025, respectively; in Liberia, the plan extends until 2021. The section assesses the implications of the density targets identified in the investment plans in relation to population

FIGURE 3.4

Concentration Curve Depicting Uneven Distribution of Health Workers, by Country

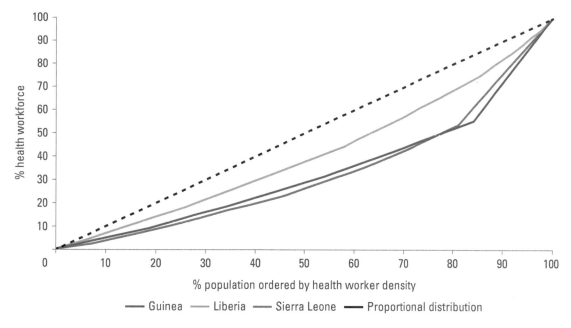

Note: This figure includes categories of health workers in the direct provision of health services (such as all categories of doctors and the nursing and midwifery workforce) and related cadres such as public health, logistics, supply chain, and laboratory services. It excludes administrative and support staff such as cleaners, maintenance, and drivers, and excludes community health volunteers.

threshold densities associated with increased service delivery coverage, graduate production, and cost.

The Investment Plans' Scaling-Up Targets

The investment plans of Guinea and Liberia mention specific health worker–to-population density targets to be achieved; this target is missing in Sierra Leone's investment plan. Liberia's stated target is 1.4 doctors, nurses, midwives, and physician assistants per 1,000 population. Removing physician assistants from this scenario produces a target density of 1.12 per 1,000 for doctors, nurses, and midwives alone. Guinea's stated target is 0.26 doctors per 1,000 population, 0.26 nurses per 1,000 population, and 0.26 midwives per 1,000 population— this produces a target density of 0.78 per 1,000 population for doctors, nurses, and midwives by 2024. In Sierra Leone's case, target densities have not been indicated in the investment plans, so the implications of using the densities proposed by the other two countries are used as a proxy in the assessments discussed below.

FIGURE 3.5
Density Targets for Doctors, Nurses, and Midwives, Compared with International Thresholds

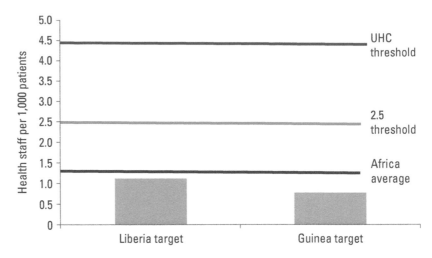

Note: UHC = universal health coverage.

The density threshold targets set in the investment plans are far below both the current regional average and international thresholds associated with improved health outcomes and service delivery indicators (figure 3.5). Commonly used international density thresholds focus on doctors, nurses, and midwives. All of the targets are substantially lower than the current regional density average of 1.33 doctors, nurses, and midwives per 1,000 population. They are also significantly lower than a commonly used workforce density threshold level of 2.5 per 1,000 population,[1] which is associated with improved service delivery coverage, as well as a new threshold of 4.45 per 1,000 population, which is associated with universal health coverage.[2] Ultimately, then, by the end of the investment plan periods, health worker densities would still be highly insufficient.

Implications of Meeting Density Targets for Scaling-Up Needs

Even the modest density targets in each investment plan translate into substantial scaling-up requirements for health workers, particularly in Guinea and Sierra Leone (table 3.2). To achieve the density targets identified in the investment plans, Liberia would have to double its number of doctors, nurses, and midwives; annual growth rates for each of the three cadres would have to be 8.2 percent to reach the proposed density targets. Guinea would have to more than triple its health workforce; Guinea's annual growth rates would have to be 15.2 percent for each cadre.

TABLE 3.2
Investment Plan Density Target Implications

Country	Implications	Doctors	Nurses	Midwives	Total
Guinea	Current stock	1,111	1,168	372	2,651
	Total stock needed to reach target density (0.78 per 1,000) in 2024 (% annual growth)	4,567 (15.2%)	4,801 (15.2%)	1,529 (15.2%)	10,897
Liberia	Current stock	158	2,445	952	3,555
	Total stock needed to reach target density (1.12 per 1,000)[a] in 2021 (% annual growth)	274 (8.2%)	4,245 (8.2%)	1,653 (8.2%)	6,172
Sierra Leone	Current stock	234	450	208	892
	Required for target density (0.78 per 1,000) in 2025 (% annual growth)	1,638 (19.4%)	3,151 (19.4%)	1,456 (19.4%)	6,244
	Required for target density (1.12 per 1,000) by 2025 (% annual growth)	2,352 (23.3%)	4,524 (23.3%)	2,091 (23.3%)	8,967

Note: a. In each case it is assumed that the current staff ratios across the three cadres will not change, so the growth rates for each cadre are the same. Note that Liberia's investment plan target has been adjusted from 1.4 per 1,000 to 1.12 per 1,000 with the removal of physician assistants for the purpose of this analysis.

If Sierra Leone were to aim to meet the same targets as Guinea and Liberia, it would have to increase its current stock more than six- to nine-fold; its annual growth rates would have to be 19.4 percent or 23.3 percent, depending on the density target chosen. It should be noted, however, that these growth rates are premised on small initial numbers. Achieving these numbers will require significantly scaling up training institution capacity as well as labor market interventions to prevent different forms of attrition.

There are significant challenges to such scaling up in terms of producing, retaining, distributing, and ensuring fiscal space that need to be considered and addressed in order to absorb a greatly expanded workforce. This is particularly important in the context of the high proportions of the current workforce not on the payroll in all three countries.

The Implication of Meeting Targets on Cost

The implication of achieving the relatively modest density targets on cost, when taking into account likely levels of attrition, is substantial. This section identifies the total and annual cost implications of the three countries pursuing their scaling-up ambitions, drawing on a number of assumptions; the total cost includes both salary and training costs, and the average salary reflected on the payroll was used. Where training cost is not known, the training cost for a staff group with similar earnings was used. Assumptions on attrition are a 10 percent workforce attrition, a 20 percent dropout rate from training, and a 50 percent employment rate in the public sector.

The annual per capita costs associated with achieving the scaling-up targets are highest in Sierra Leone, followed by Liberia; they are substantially lower in Guinea. In Sierra Leone, achieving a target similar to Guinea's in 2024 would cost US$18.25 per capita annually; achieving a target similar to Liberia's in 2024 would cost US$24.10 per capita annually. In Liberia, when taking into account attrition, achieving the proposed target of 1.12 nurses, midwives, and physicians per 1,000 population in 2021 would cost US$8.19 per capita annually. In Guinea, achieving the proposed target of 0.78 nurses, midwives, and physicians per 1,000 population in 2024 would cost US$1.51 per capita annually. Table 3.3 provides the total annual cost implications for each country to achieve its respective density scaling-up targets.

The large variation in cost raises questions about the observed differences in per capita costs and training costs needed to secure quality training programs and motivated staff committed to public sector work. Although levels are not expressed in purchasing-power-parity terms, the differences are too large to be fully accounted for by any differences in the value of the U.S. dollar in each setting. Note that costing data were not available for Sierra Leone, so regional values were used as proxies, and thus may not reflect the actual costs of workforce production in Sierra Leone. Further data gathering and analysis for Sierra Leone are therefore warranted.

TABLE 3.3
Total Annual Cost Implications of Scaling Up Needed to Reach Investment Plan Density Targets
U.S. dollars

Country	Annual cost	Doctors	Nurses	Midwives	Total cost
Guinea	Annual cost in 2024	10,714,901	7,789,027	2,629,596	21,133,524
Liberia	Annual cost in 2021	7,893,628	29,004,044	8,277,607	45,175,279
Sierra Leone	Annual cost in 2024 target density similar to Liberia's of 1.12/1,000	124,285,019	50,227,855	14,706,974	189,219,848
	Annual cost in 2024 target density similar to Guinea's of 0.78/1,000	94,252,971	37,997,117	11,011,779	143,261,866

Note: The years represent the end points of the investment plans. The length of the investment plan timeline is important to consider when making training cost comparisons. The longer it takes to reach the target density, the more health workers will be lost to attrition and the more trainees will be required. Cost implications exclude inflation.

Scaling Up Needed to Meet Global Density Thresholds

The previous section has shown the investment plan density targets are nowhere near the health worker–to–population ratios associated with sufficient service delivery coverage and health outcomes. This section assesses the scaling up needed for each country to reach the international threshold of 2.5 doctors, nurses, and midwives per 1,000 population and discusses the implications of this scaling up for the number of graduates needed (taking into account different forms of attrition) and the cost of reaching this threshold.

Implications of Health Worker Scaling Up for Meeting Global Thresholds

The number of health workers needed to meet the international threshold of 2.5 doctors, nurses, and midwives per 1,000 population is a lot higher than envisioned in the investment plans. Table 3.4 shows the current numbers of doctors, nurses, and midwives in each country and how many will be required to achieve 2.5 per 1,000 population overall density by the years 2020, 2025, and 2030; the table assumes a continuation of the current ratios of staff across the three cadres. Years 2020, 2025, and 2030 were used instead of the actual plan dates of 2021, 2024, and 2025 because they are seen as more realistic years for achieving the thresholds.

The annual growth rates required for each threshold date and each country are much higher than those required to meet the density targets currently set out in the investment plans or derived from the costing tool (table 3.5). However, setting a later target date of 2030

TABLE 3.4

Number of Workers Required to Meet 2.5 per 1,000 Population Density, by 2020, 2025, and 2030

Stock	Guinea			Liberia			Sierra Leone		
	Doctors	Nurses	Midwives	Doctors	Nurses	Midwives	Doctors	Nurses	Midwives
Current stock	1,111	1,168	372	158	2,445	952	234	450	208
Total required in 2020	13,108	13,781	4,389	593	9,184	3,576	4,754	9,142	4,225
Total required in 2025	15,049	15,821	5,039	699	10,814	4,211	5,251	10,098	4,668
Total required in 2030	17,312	18,200	5,797	824	12,748	4,964	5,804	11,162	5,159

TABLE 3.5
Growth Rates Required to Achieve Different Targets, by Target Dates
Annual percent

Country	Growth rate of doctors, nurses, and midwives		
	To reach international norms	To reach density thresholds of investment plan	To reach costing plan targets (see appendix B.2)
Guinea	50.1% (2020); 26.7% (2025); 18.7% (2030)	15.2% (2024)	14.3% (2024)
Liberia	24.7% (2020); 14.5% (2025); 10.9% (2030)	9.7% (2021)	10.3% (2021)
Sierra Leone	65.2% (2020); 32.7% (2025); 22.2% (2030)	19.4%–23.3% (2025)	9% (2025)

requires only slightly higher rates of growth than those required by the investment plans.

Applying these annual growth rates, and a target date of 2030, Guinea's scaling-up requirements are the largest of the three countries to achieve the 2.5 doctors, nurses, and midwives per 1,000 threshold. Figure 3.6 shows the workforce scaling up needed over the 2015 to 2030 period for doctors, nurses, and midwives in each country. Given the high levels of the growth rates required to achieve targets in 2020 and 2025, especially in Guinea and Sierra Leone, the following analyses assume a 2030 target date for achieving the required workforce scaling up as a more realistic goal, and one that is comparable across the three countries.

Implications of Meeting Global Density Thresholds for Graduate Production

Moving on to estimate the number of graduates needed requires taking into account different forms of attrition. Given the absence of robust comparable data on workforce attrition, training dropout rates, and employment rates, theoretical scenarios on attrition were generated that take these variables into account.

When different forms of attrition, dropout rates, and employment rates, are taken into account, the number of annual graduates required to meet scaling-up targets is much higher than the estimated total growth in numbers. Figure 3.7 shows the estimated number of graduates required to meet the international threshold of 2.5 per 1,000 population when one of the scenarios on attrition is applied. It shows that Guinea's

FIGURE 3.6

Workforce (Doctors, Nurses, and Midwives) Scaling Up Needed to Reach the International Threshold, 2014–30

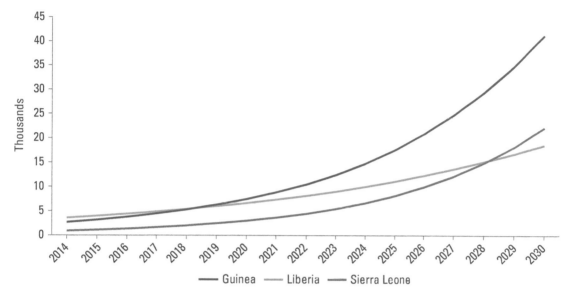

Note: The analysis in this figure applies the growth rate needed to achieve the proposed target by 2030.

FIGURE 3.7

Numbers of Trainees (Doctors, Nurses, and Midwives) Needed to Reach the International Threshold, 2015–29

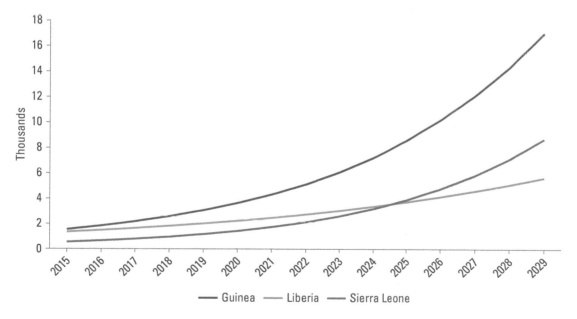

Note: The analysis presented in this figure applies the growth rate needed to achieve the proposed target by 2030.

scaling up would have to be the steepest. In the figure, scaling up is based on a scenario in which attrition from the workforce is 10 percent (the average graduate who takes up health sector employment works for 10 years in the role), dropout from training is 20 percent, and 50 percent of graduates take up employment in the (public) health sector.

When taking into account attrition, the vast challenges the three countries face in scaling up their workforces to reach acceptable densities is highlighted. All three countries currently struggle to produce even current levels of graduate output and are fighting to contain current labor market inefficiencies, causing attrition and flow to other sectors. Far more international support is needed for the three countries to address their current training capacity weaknesses, as well as existing market inefficiencies, if acceptable levels of health workers are to be produced. Furthermore, as highlighted in the sections below, emphasis needs to be placed on training and deploying the health workforce into underserved areas for primary health care.

Implications of Meeting Global Thresholds for Cost

This section provides an overview of the costs that it will require each of the three countries to achieve the international thresholds by 2030, when taking into account three different scenarios of attrition (table 3.6). As applied above, some assumptions used in the cost projections are total costs, which include salary and training costs; the average salary reflected on the payroll was used; and where the training cost is not known, the training cost for a staff group with similar earnings was used.

Applying different levels of attrition, training dropout rates, and employment rates, the three countries differ markedly in what it will cost per capita to achieve the same workforce density by 2030. Table 3.7 projects the total costs for achieving minimum recommended workforce densities under Scenario 2 and the alternative scenario of 5 percent attrition, a 10 percent dropout rate from training, and a 75 percent uptake of the relevant health

TABLE 3.6
Theoretical Scenarios of Attrition and Employment
Percent

Scenario	Workforce attrition	Drop out of training	Employment rate
Base scenario	0	0	100
Scenario 1	5	10	75
Scenario 2	10	20	50

TABLE 3.7
Cost of Achieving Minimum Densities of Doctors, Nurses, and Midwives, 2015–29, under Two Scenarios
U.S. dollars, millions/cost per capita

Country	Scenario	2015	2020	2025	2029
Guinea	Scenario 2	6.7/0.6	15.8/1.3	37.4/2.6	74.3/4.6
	Scenario 1	6.1/0.6	14.3/1.1	33.7/2.3	67.0/4.2
Liberia	Scenario 2	16.2/3.6	27.2/5.1	5.6/7.3	68.9/9.6
	Scenario 1	13.3/2.9	22.3/4.2	37.4/5.9	56.5/7.9
Sierra Leone	Scenario 2	27.8/4.2	75.9/10.5	207.2/25.9	462.3/53.3
	Scenario 1	23.7/3.6	64.6/8.9	176.2/22.0	393.3/45.3

professional role in the health sector by graduates (Scenario 1). Table 3.7 shows that this cost ranges from US$4.2 per capita in Guinea, Scenario 1, to US$53.3 per capita in Sierra Leone, Scenario 2, in 2029 (the last year in which trainees graduate to achieve the 2030 target).

The differences across countries reflect large differences in cost estimates for wages and for training (figure 3.8). These differences are far more important in the overall cost projection than the scenario differences that in each case halve attrition, dropping out from training, and losses from graduates not taking up public sector employment, suggesting that priority attention to right-sizing cost levels is needed and ensuring that the estimates used in this analysis are accurate. Variation in salaries accounts for major differences—for example, in Guinea the costs are estimated at about US$1,200 for a doctor's salary per year and US$2,800 to train a doctor, respectively. Based on higher regional production cost estimates and salary schemes in Sierra Leone (in light of the many health workers being trained abroad), the cost of a doctor in the labor force is nearly US$16,000 and training a doctor is estimated at US$100,000 (local data were not available at the time of the analysis, so estimates should be interpreted with some caution).

Although the totals required for scaling up in Guinea and Liberia might be affordable, it is unlikely that Sierra Leone will be able to allocate US$50 per capita for a workforce of doctors, nurses, and midwives. Reducing costs of doctors or concentrating on scaling up the availability of nurses and midwives would make a significant difference. For example, if the density of 2.5 per 1,000 population were achieved by scaling up only nurses and midwives, the 2029 cost would fall to US$22 per capita for Scenario 1. This is still high compared with the cost for Guinea or

FIGURE 3.8

Estimated Annual Costs for Health Workforce (Doctors, Nurses, and Midwives) plus Training Costs

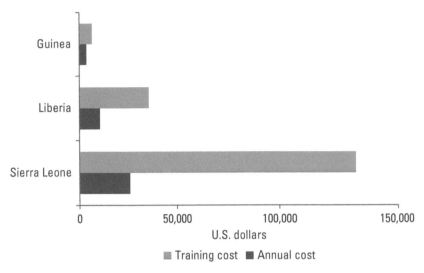

Note: Based on regional training cost estimates for Sierra Leone.

Liberia because of the still relatively high estimated training costs of nurses and midwives in Sierra Leone.

Guinea's costs are low because of the low estimated wage bill and because of the lower training costs in that country. These are likely to be unrealistically low, in the sense that they may not secure adequate training quality or adequate motivation to work effectively in the public sector. If Guinea is to achieve effective access to services for its population, it may need to increase its public sector pay rates for both clinical workers themselves and for those working in training institutions. Guinea may also need to ensure that other requirements of training—related to the sufficient physical, technical, and organizational capacities of health training institutions—are adequately resourced.

How Do Scaling-Up Plans Fit into the Projected Picture on Fiscal Space in the Three Countries?

Ambitions related to achieving so-called needs-based indicators founded on achieving international thresholds should be treated with caution. Ultimately, a country should and will produce only as many health workers as it can afford to train and absorb. A focus on forecasting that takes into account the overall fiscal space available to absorb costs is thus critical. This section looks at the extent to which the fiscal space for HRH (current and projected) is sufficient to accommodate the proposed scaling up and potential scaling up to internationally recommended density targets. It draws on the same assumptions and data as the overall fiscal space analysis in chapter 5, but teases out HRH in particular.

Table B.1.2 (in appendix B.1) shows different cost projections reanalyzed to a common future point (2020). GDP and government expenditures have been estimated for 2020 based on IMF projections (as of April 2016). Further projection to 2030 compares a pessimistic scenario (no growth in these indicators between 2020 and 2030) and a more optimistic scenario (5 percent annual growth in these indicators between 2020 and 2030).

Based on the national investment plans, all countries project a declining proportion of total health expenditures accounted for by the wage bill. However, if Sierra Leone were to attempt to achieve Guinea's desired ratio of doctors, nurses, and midwives of 0.78 per 1,000 population, this would result in an increasing share of total health expenditures being absorbed by workforce costs, from the current level of about 51 percent to 182 percent. These higher levels of cost in Sierra Leone reflect high costs in general in the country, particularly high training costs and high costs of doctors (with many trained abroad), which, as discussed, need to be interpreted with caution. Much lower costs and shares of expenditures for achieving the same density target, along with other planned health workforce increases in Guinea, reflect the low pay and training costs in that country as well as its relatively unambitious scaling-up plans given the projected health expenditure increase.

In Guinea and Liberia, projected fiscal space seems to be adequate to accommodate the proposed scaling-up and density targets outlined in the investment plans, although this should be interpreted with caution. The conclusion to be drawn from figure 3.9 is that projected fiscal space in Guinea and Liberia appears sufficient to support the absorption of investment plan target densities. As mentioned above, this cannot be said about Sierra Leone. At the same time, these densities reflect the levels of doctors, nurses, and midwives only, and do not include all the other cadres that need to be accommodated by the public sector wage bill. Furthermore, any fiscal space projections are highly contingent on the accuracy of the projected GDP rates and public and health expenditure levels.

With the similar exception of Sierra Leone, the fiscal space needed to reach international thresholds also appears to be sufficient, although again caution is necessary. The projection of the costs associated with the ambition of achieving international doctor, nurse, and midwife density thresholds of 2.5 per 1,000 population by 2030 increases the projected share of health workforce costs in total health expenditure costs considerably, but to shares that would not be outliers by international standards in Guinea and Liberia, even if no further growth in health budgets is projected after 2020 (see figure 3.9). Sierra Leone seems to be the outlier, and could not achieve this target at its current estimated cost levels, even if further growth in health budgets is projected at 5 percent per annum from 2020 to 2030. At the same time, again, these scaling-up projections and related costs reflect only doctors, nurses, and midwives, and do not

FIGURE 3.9
Wage Bill as a Proportion of Health Expenditures under Different Cost Projections

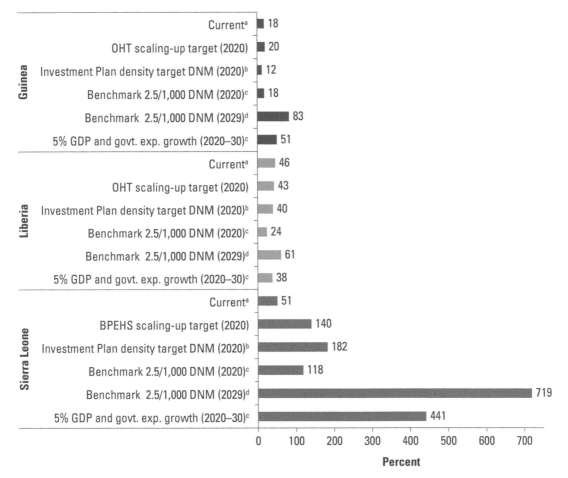

Source: International Monetary Fund, World Economic Outlook Database, April 2016.
Note: This is a summary table based on calculations in table B.1.2 in appendix B.1. BPEHS = Basic Package of Essential Health Services; DNM = doctors, nurses, and midwives; OHT = One Health Tool.
a. Current estimates are based on 2016 cost projections compared to 2014 levels of GDP, total government expenditures, and government expenditures on health using government expenditures on health as a percentage of total government expenditures: 3.67 percent for Guinea, 12.4 percent for Liberia, and 7.1 percent for Sierra Leone. Estimates for 2020 are calculated using target percentages discussed in government fiscal space publications.
b. As per density targets for doctors, nurses, and midwives in country investment plans (Sierra Leone's projection uses the 0.78/1,000 population density target).
c. Total cost estimates for doctors, nurses, and midwives represent those in progress toward target 2020 and 2029.
For 2.5/1,000 population projection, the target date used is 2030.
d. 2020 national data projections.

take into account all other cadres that will need to be accommodated and absorbed by the wage bill.

Moreover, unless effective measures are put in place to tackle different forms of attrition, fiscal space scenarios may be insufficient. Even though the least-ambitious scenario for attrition, dropping out, and employment has been used in the fiscal space analysis, real current rates may be even higher than these, suggesting that no scenario may be sustainable unless effective measures are put in place to tackle these problems. Tension is likely to exist between controlling cost levels and controlling attrition, dropout, and employment losses to the health workforce.

Overall, when taking into account all health workers, projected fiscal space is likely to be insufficient for all three countries. Although reaching scaling-up targets and international thresholds of doctors, nurses, and midwives seemingly could be accommodated in Guinea and Liberia (albeit not in Sierra Leone), it should be noted that they represent only around 30 percent of the total health workforce in Liberia, 37 percent in Guinea, and 8 percent in Sierra Leone. While a more comprehensive analysis of scaling-up projections for all cadres and fiscal space absorption capacity was not in the scope of this book, it is clear that reaching the doctors, nurses, and midwives targets and thresholds *in addition to* accommodating existing numbers and scaling up other health cadres is probably not fiscally feasible. Accommodating a density of doctors, nurses, and midwives of 2.5/1,000 in Guinea by 2029 alone would require a wage bill of 83 percent of total health expenditures (and in Liberia, 61 percent). As such, and as emphasized in the following section on distribution, each country may need to focus on scaling up lower-level cadres who are cheaper to train and employ, and who are more likely to take up employment in rural and remote areas (where most of the population live).

Health Workforce Distribution: Investment Plan Strategies

Although all three investment plans address the issue of distribution, Liberia's plan provides the greatest amount of detail. The Liberia investment plan specifies a housing allowance for 10 percent of the workforce (in underserved areas) and plans to develop fair and equitable remuneration by introducing and financing a hardship allowance, among other things. Guinea's and Sierra Leone's plans discuss the aim of establishing an effective system of incentives and allocation of staff to underserved areas, but actual strategies in their plans are not currently defined. Both countries, however, point to the importance of carrying out labor market assessments in order to identify strategies that target solutions to address rural/urban imbalances, which is a positive step. Moreover, both Liberia and Sierra Leone specifically emphasize the importance of developing a community health worker (CHW) program (discussed further below) with the specific objective of ensuring greater health worker coverage in rural areas. Although not specifically discussed in its own plan, Guinea has similar ambitions.

Sufficient emphasis on the urban/rural distribution issue will be critical because the vast majority of the population in all three countries will continue to live in rural areas. Although urban populations are projected to increase slightly faster, proportional to rural populations, the majority will continue to live in rural areas. Figure 3.10 shows the rural and urban population projections through 2029 for Sierra Leone. The picture is similar in the other two countries.

Reaching the density targets stated in the investment plans would require significantly larger growth rates of health workers for rural areas, particularly in Guinea and Sierra Leone. Although requirements in urban areas are moderate in all cases, the high urban/rural disparities in Guinea and Sierra Leone imply that very high rates of growth for rural employed health workers will be needed to achieve targets in these areas. The low base for some of the projections—for example, currently Guinea has only 22 rural doctors—drives the high growth rates calculated. This analysis highlights the urgent need for countries to focus on addressing workforce

FIGURE 3.10
Rural and Urban Population Projections, 2014–30: Example of Sierra Leone

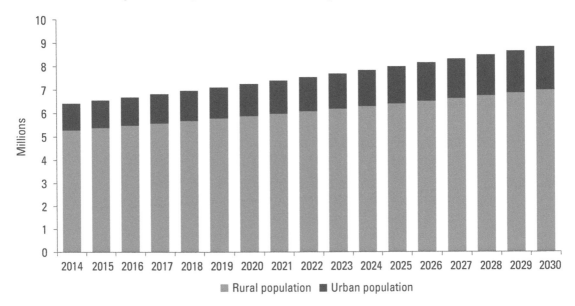

TABLE 3.8
Annual Rural versus Urban Growth Rates Required to Reach Plan Targets
Percent

Country (target year)	Doctors		Nurses		Midwives	
	Urban	Rural	Urban	Rural	Urban	Rural
Guinea (2024)	11.3	63.0	12.3	33.7	11.5	44.3
Liberia (2021)	5.6	12.2	6.0	6.9	6.1	2.4
Sierra Leone (2025)	4.2	49.9	6.8	33.8	6.8	34.3

distribution in their scaling-up plans. Table 3.8 shows the workforce growth rates required for plan targets in each country, broken down by rural and urban requirements.

If current rural/urban ratios are kept constant, a worsening of the rural/urban imbalance in Guinea and Sierra Leone would be expected; this would not be as severe in Liberia. Keeping rural/urban ratios of cadres constant (taking into account the projected numbers of doctors, nurses, and midwives), and assuming no additional interventions or external influences that affect rural labor market uptake, health worker densities in rural areas would improve only very minimally in all three countries, although disproportionately so in urban areas (figure 3.11). Whereas the rural/urban distribution would improve in Liberia under these assumptions, in Guinea and Sierra Leone it would worsen considerably (given the already greater rural incentives in place for doctors, nurses, and midwives relative to the other two countries).

The fairly strong emphasis on scaling up higher-level cadres in all three countries may do little to improve already high rural/urban disparities. The assessment of the cadre-specific targets outlined in the costing exercise that accompanied these plans (appendix B.2 includes this assessment) shows that all three countries emphasize the scaling up of high-level cadres and have varying degrees of emphasis on scaling up mid- and lower-level cadres. Guinea's greatest emphasis is mid-level workers (nurses and midwives), though high-level workers (physicians) are also a focus. Liberia is emphasizing the scaling up of high-level worker cadres (physicians) and midwives. Sierra Leone is focusing on the scaling up of high-level workers (general practitioners and specialists) as well as some low-level cadres (nurse and midwife associates, medical and laboratory lab technicians). When not combined with effective policies that foster rural labor market uptake of health professionals (there is less evidence that incentive policies can achieve this than rural pipeline policies),

FIGURE 3.11
Density of Health Workers (Doctors, Nurses, and Midwives) per 1,000 Population in Rural and Urban Areas, 2014 and Projected

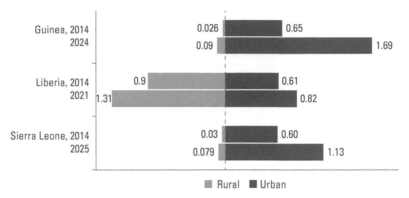

Note: Projected health worker density assumes no changes to the current status quo. It uses cadre targets as outlined in the costing tools and assumes that the distribution of health workers of each cadre between rural and urban areas remains the same over time. This figure assumes that no policies or programs for redistribution are implemented, and that the rural/urban distribution of the workforce will not be influenced by the absolute number of health workers, relative population growth, or health worker density.

This figure assumes that no policies or programs for redistribution are implemented, and that the rural/urban distribution of the workforce will not be influenced by the absolute number of health workers, relative population growth, or health worker density.

high- and mid-level cadres tend to be much more unevenly distributed than lower-level ones (see figure 3.12).

In this regard, the emphasis on CHWs, when adequately trained and integrated into the existing health system, may be able to improve accessibility to some health services in rural areas, but may not be sufficient. Investment plans in all three countries do propose reforms and scaling-up plans for community health volunteers (CHVs) and CHWs. There are important differences in the nature of existing and planned CHVs and CHWs across the three countries.

In 2016, **Guinea** will accelerate the implementation of the community health plan with the decision to further train technical health officers (agents technique de santé, or ATSs) to become CHWs. Guinea has a large number of ATSs (4,284) already working at the peripheral level and paid by the government (the ATS is a formalized cadre on the payroll). This model is notable in that it reflects a rural pipeline approach and the institutionalization of the training of CHWs in the health system. In addition, Guinea has a large number of CHVs who also support health services provision (43,000). Evidence of the value of sporadic training of CHVs, without adequately integrating them into the health system, is very limited.

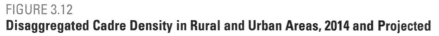

FIGURE 3.12

Disaggregated Cadre Density in Rural and Urban Areas, 2014 and Projected

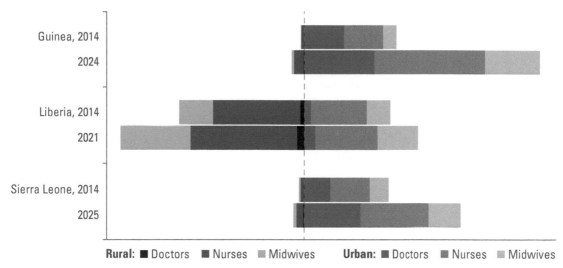

Note: Projected health worker density uses cadre targets as outlined in the costing tools and assumes that the distribution of health workers of each cadre between rural and urban areas remains the same over time.

According to a 2013 mapping exercise in **Liberia**, there were over 8,000 CHVs of various types (for example, general CHVs, trained traditional midwives, and community health support groups such as household health promoters, community-directed distributors, mass drug distributors, and community-based distributors). These CHVs are not on the payroll, though they have been mobilized and incentivized to varying extents for service provision and public health campaigns by various health programs. They played an important role throughout the Ebola response. The investment plan and a new CHW policy propose establishing a new cadre of formalized CHWs with a standard package of training to provide a standard package of services. A total of 4,100 CHWs will be trained and deployed over five years to provide services to a population of 1.2 million people who live more than 5 kilometers from a health facility. These CHWs will be selected from, although not limited to, the existing pool of CHVs. CHWs will be paid though a performance-based incentive, mostly by donor-funded schemes. Although not fully integrated into the existing scheme, this strategy could be promising.

In **Sierra Leone**, there has been significant interest in and attention to the use of CHWs. However, existing CHWs (not on the payroll) currently deployed differ widely in their skills and abilities, and are not adequately integrated into the existing health system. There are estimated to be 10,000 to 15,000 CHWs in Sierra Leone. Existing training for CHWs is around 10 days; this category is often considered to be analogous to CHVs in other countries. The CHW strategic policy in Sierra Leone is currently under discussion and review.

Planning for community-based cadres should be integrated into broader health workforce planning. It is critical not to see CHWs and CHVs in isolation, ignoring the fact that these cadres—even when sufficiently trained and remunerated and integrated into the system—require a wider complementarity and the support structure of other health workers (including doctors, physician assistants, nurses, midwives, health assistants, and other cadres) and links with other levels of care. Working together as a team, health workers can deliver services to the populations at the periphery of the health system.

Discussion and Conclusions

The analysis presented in this chapter provides a better understanding of the implications of the investment plans and costing exercises for scaling-up ambitions. Data are largely based on public payroll data, which are limited, and the analysis is based on crude theoretical scenarios. At the same time, a number of key conclusions and recommendations can be drawn, which are noted below, and are presented in greater detail in chapter 5.

Reaching the targets identified in the investment plans (and the accompanying costing exercises) will not substantially improve health worker densities, particularly in Guinea and Sierra Leone. When population growth rates are taken into account, the health worker–to–population ratio that will result from achieving the set targets will remain far below the current regional average and even further behind international thresholds for decades to come.

From a fiscal perspective, both Guinea and Liberia could accommodate meeting the conservative scaling-up targets in their investment plans as well as the international thresholds, although they focus on doctors, nurses, and midwives only. The calculations provided in the report have shown that the costs associated with reaching the investment plan targets as well as the more ambitious international thresholds (for example, the 2.5 doctors, nurses, and midwives per 1,000 population density) could largely be accommodated by the fiscal space projections around HRH, except in Sierra Leone, where training costs of health workers seem to be substantially higher than they are in the other two countries (stemming in part from the cost of training doctors abroad, which is a necessity given the current state of the medical education system). At the same time, the targets and thresholds focus on doctors, nurses, and midwives alone, and so do not represent the entire health workforce.

Projected fiscal space in all three countries is likely to be insufficient when taking into account all other health worker cadres on the public payroll. Although investment plan targets and international threshold densities are limited to doctors, nurses, and midwives only, this group as a share of the total health workforce (on the public payroll) is relatively small: 37 percent in Guinea, 30 percent in Liberia, and 8 percent in Sierra Leone. Although a detailed analysis of the scaling-up costs for all health cadres was not possible, the findings of the report indicate that projected fiscal space would be stretched considerably more when all other health cadres are included. This suggests that actually reaching the doctor, nurse, and midwife density targets as outlined in some of the investment plans, as well as reaching higher international thresholds, would not only have a limited impact on health worker to population densities but would also not be financially feasible.

Efforts to reach target densities and international thresholds, moreover, would be constrained by the limited production capacity in each of the three countries. Particularly when different forms of attrition are taken into consideration, to reach even the relatively modest targets currently outlined in the investment plans would require stretching the capacity to produce this output far more in all three countries than perhaps anticipated. The extent to which each country could consider boosting its ambitions and aim to achieve more ambitious benchmarks would stretch this capacity even further. What is more important, however, and is discussed further below, is that such training and scaling up cannot follow the traditional models of training if it is to achieve its desired impact.

To address prevailing needs within a constrained fiscal space scenario, a paradigm shift in *who* to train and *how* to train health workers is needed in all three countries. The biggest challenge in all countries is not the lack of health workers available at the aggregate level, but the staggering shortage of health workers available in rural areas. This is where the vast majority of the population live (and will continue to live), and where maternal and child health outcomes are disproportionately poor. Inaction and maintaining the existing skill mix currently being produced is likely to preserve rural/urban disparities as they are now—an issue that is extremely problematic in all countries, although slightly better in Liberia. A greater emphasis on scaling up (urban-trained) higher-level cadres is not just expensive, but is also likely to further worsen the rural/urban distribution of health workers, with global evidence showing that higher-level cadres, trained and used to living in urban areas (including moonlighting in the private sector), are less likely to take up rural posts than health workers with opposite traits.

While high-level cadres and urban training environments play an important role in each of these countries—in particular to meet faculty needs, secondary- and tertiary-level service delivery needs, and private sector demand—public sector investments should prioritize the production of health workers with the greatest social rates of return, focusing on competencies needed for UHC and ensuring their presence in parts of the country where needs are greatest. Consideration should be given as to the role of the private sector in the training of higher-level cadres in each of the three countries.

To make a real impact, the public sector focus needs to be primarily on innovative training policies to scale up the rural health workforce. When *combined* with country- and cadre-specific monetary and nonmonetary incentive policies, such policies hold the potential to address many of the concerns related to HRH in all three countries. The specifics of these policies will vary from country to country and from health worker to health worker. *Rural pipeline policies* refer to decentralized training approaches where health workers *from* rural areas are trained *in* rural areas and *for* rural areas, and provided with the continuous support, supervision, and mentorship needed to ensure retention. The logic is that health workers who are familiar with rural surroundings and tied to their friends and families there are much more likely to work in such environments upon graduation than their urban counterparts. Some common examples of such programs are highlighted in box 3.1.

Such strategies should be combined with a focus on training lower- and mid-level cadres for rural service; they are not only cheaper to train, but are also linked to increased rural employment uptake and retention.

BOX 3.1
Global Examples of Training and Incentive Programs for a Rural Health Workforce

A few countries have developed specific approaches to training a rural workforce and to developing appropriate incentive policies. Liberia, for example, has made rural rotations of its postgraduate medical education professionals mandatory. Ethiopia developed a health extension program (where workers selected from rural areas are trained in and for rural areas), which is comparable in size and ambition to the effective and well-documented family health program in Brazil. Thailand's program of developing a pipeline of rural doctors reinforced by monetary incentives is emulated by South Africa and Canada (with the Northern School of Ontario – Canada). Uganda's Makerere University introduced a new Family Health Physician program as an incentive for rural-based family practice, combining specialization and rural workforce needs, as did Sudan at its Gezira University. While all these are popular examples and have expanded the rural health workforce, none of these programs is without its challenges, and any new program should be closely linked to contuinuous assessment and impact evaluation.

Low- and mid-level cadres—such as auxiliary workers, health assistants, and technologists—tend to be more willing to work in rural areas than higher-level cadres. With additional training and support, such cadres have the potential to be just as or more effective than higher-level cadres in performing primary care services, yet take shorter times to train and have higher rates of social return. Mid-level cadres—such as physician assistants, nurses, and midwifes in Liberia—can also be effectively deployed and retained in rural areas, provided they are better incentivized to work in rural areas and are appropriately supported. Mid-level cadres could also be rapidly trained to take on advanced roles, such as nurses and physician assistants trained as anesthetists, ophthalmic nurses, or mental health clinicians in Liberia. Furthermore, the production of alternative cadres specific only to the country is a promising strategy often combined with a rural pipeline approach. Cadres (such as physician assistants, non-clinician physicians) who are specifically trained for rural service and are less competitive in the national (urban/private market) and international labor markets should also be further explored. Such strategies, which seem to be globally promising, require support from various medical, nursing, and midwifery associations. In several of these countries such cadres already exist; for example, agents technique de santé (ATS) in Guinea and physician assistants in Liberia could be further scaled up and provided with additional support.

The emphasis on CHW scaling up in all three countries is notable, but should be carefully considered and not seen as an end in itself. There is little evidence that CHWs (many of them volunteers), when sporadically trained and not adequately integrated into a frontline health worker team and the wider health system, can have a sufficient impact on health outcomes. CHWs should thus not be seen in isolation as a solution; the emphasis on their integration and connectedness (and acceptance) with other health workers is an important yet challenging one. Any efforts to scale up CHW programs should be carefully considered and designed, slowly rolled out, and monitored throughout prior to larger scaling-up ambitions. Plans for CHV and CHW development should be integrated into a broader health workforce design and require further evidence-based analysis and policy dialogue to ensure that such programs take a labor market perspective and represent the most efficient investment in workforce development to achieve health goals.

Any training efforts toward a fit-for-purpose health workforce should be combined with a continued focus on ensuring and improving capacities related to health worker performance. Numbers alone do not guarantee effective and sufficient service delivery outcomes, and health workers—particularly in rural areas—often exhibit low performance standards. The type of performance constraint needs to be carefully identified and tends to differ by cadre, location, and sector. Assessments should be carried out to identify potential gaps in competencies related to maternal and child health service delivery, as well as those related to disease surveillance and response (see box 3.2). Suboptimal performance also arises from a number of factors beyond those related to training and knowledge. These factors include the lack of adequate supplies and motivation. Here, too, assessments should be carried out to identify existing constraints. Overall, health worker performance should be understood to be a function of both capacity (supplies, knowledge) and effort (motivation), and weaknesses and solutions should be identified for each.

While efforts to train an appropriate skill mix for UHC will yield improvements over the medium to long terms, this should be coupled with short-term capacity-building measures for existing health workers at all levels of the health system. Such measures are already in place in some countries and may require scaling up. Standardized, team-based short-term training programs and approaches, strengthened mentoring and opportunities for continuous professional development, and effective supportive supervision coupled with clearly defined referral structures and professional scopes of practice are all critical for success. In addition, such strategies should also be reinforced with monetary and non-monetary incentives, as appropriate, when these are based on evidence from health labor market assessments.

For all three countries, the specific interventions required to implement their investment plans should be guided by rigorous health education and health labor market assessments. Evidence is critical and needed, both from well-designed and repeated health training institution assessments in order to identify existing capacity constraints, and from health labor market assessments in order to identify the factors that

---

BOX 3.2
Strengthening the Health Workforce for Disease Surveillance and Response

In all three countries, the lack of health workers and a weak capacity to respond to the crisis was a central reason that Ebola spun out of control. To minimize a recurrence, a significant strengthening of the health workforce, as argued throughout this chapter, is necessary. And what is needed is not to scale up particular cadres for the delivery of vertical health programs, but instead an effort to horizontally strengthen the competencies of health workers across all levels of the health system, from the community level upward, integrating disease surveillance and response elements into existing maternal and child health training programs. Such capacity building, in the form of strengthening existing curricula and/or providing relevant in-service training and mentoring to address existing weaknesses, needs to be guided and informed by regular and rigorous competency assessments of health workers across all levels of the system.

motivate health workers to seek employment or perform better in a particular sector, type of health facility, or geographic location. Such assessments and evidence are absolutely essential to the design of targeted and effective policies that address prevailing problems. The mention of the importance of such studies in the investment plans of all three countries, in particular health labor market assessments, is a step in the right direction on this issue and needs to be supported by the World Bank immediately. This can be followed by collaborative efforts between the World Bank's Health and Education Department to consider relevant, strategically practical investments.

Notes

1. A threshold of 2.28 doctors, nurses, and midwives per 1,000 population has been globally associated with 80 percent of skilled birth attendance coverage. Subsequent calculations using updated data, as well as the calculation of relationships between health worker densities and vaccination coverage, have revealed this desired density threshold to be slightly higher. Therefore, a rounded-up ratio of 2.5 was used to take this into account.
2. This is a new threshold, as first reported by the World Health Organization, *Global Strategy on Human Resources for Health: Workforce 2030*, http://who.int /hrh/resources/globstrathrh-2030/en/.

CHAPTER 4

Scaling Up the Disease Surveillance System

Introduction

The focus of this chapter is to lay the analytical foundation for regional disease surveillance and response (RDSR) networks, which are founded on effective national systems. It first establishes the reason that disease surveillance systems are essential to health systems strengthening at the national level, and then makes the investment case for establishing an integrated RDSR network in West Africa. The chapter then looks briefly at the methodology used to determine the value-added benefits of an RDSR, reviews best practices adopted for existing surveillance systems through case studies of successful networks, and lays out the elements that are essential for an effective and efficient network. The final sections consider the operational and fixed costs of an RDSR network and requirements for its sustainability.

A core priority under the health systems strengthening investment plans is to strengthen disease surveillance systems *within* each country. For Guinea, improving the health information system and strengthening the prevention and management of diseases and emergency situations is listed as a priority pillar under the Guinea Health Development Plan (2015–24). The Government of Liberia has identified the need to strengthen epidemic preparedness, surveillance, and response as a key priority area under the Liberia Health System Strengthening Investment Plan (2015–21). Similarly, a priority pillar under the Sierra Leone Health Sector Recovery Plan (2015–20) is to improve the information system and surveillance capacity and to implement all eight core capacities of the International Health Regulations (IHR) (2005) during the long-term recovery phase. Country plans for enhancing the surveillance, preparedness, and response capacities of the health system are generally inward looking; they do not adequately address the transboundary nature of infectious disease outbreaks, and they provide insufficient attention to cross-sector and cross-border collaboration. Although the bulk of investment in a functional disease surveillance network must be directed toward improving national and subnational capacity, there is a need for complementary marginal investment in regional network functions to ensure collaboration, information sharing, and collective action in the face of a disease threat.

The benefits of investing in an RDSR network in West Africa lie first and foremost in the global public good nature of such an investment: when infectious disease outbreaks are left undetected or detected late, they are more likely to spread rapidly to other neighboring countries, and mitigation costs grow exponentially because of delays in detection brought about by systemic weaknesses. The presence of an RDSR network in the subregion will help address these weaknesses, and the benefits of regional networking arrangements are bound to accrue to all member countries. Additionally, the establishment of an RDSR network can promote regional cooperation and better coordination in the sharing of resources among member countries. This results in better economies of scale and efficiency gains in the implementation of country core capacities in resource-limited settings for effective disease surveillance and response, in line with the WHO International Health Regulations (IHR 2005).[1,2]

As evidenced by the 2014 epidemic of Ebola virus disease (EVD) in Guinea, Liberia, and Sierra Leone, which resulted in an estimated forgone output of approximately US$1.6 billion combined (UNDG 2015), highly contagious diseases in this region cross borders easily and have the potential to turn into pandemics. The most recent outbreak of Zika virus, which is spreading rapidly across the Latin America and the Caribbean region (and at the time of this report, was threatening to spread into parts of the southern United States), and is expected to have an economic impact currently estimated at US$3.5 billion in 2016, is another reminder of the increasing interconnectedness of countries within and across regions. Results from a Markov Chain Monte Carlo simulation model show the average loss to the West African regional economy from the occurrence of a pandemic to be estimated at US$12 billion per year.[3] The fluid nature of infectious disease outbreaks across countries, which have the potential to turn into large-scale epidemics or pandemics, dramatically illustrates the need for a more harmonized and coordinated approach to disease surveillance, preparedness, and response, and the need to put in place better early warning systems and other proactive methods for preventing and controlling infectious disease outbreaks in the subregion. This need underscores the importance of regional cooperation among West African countries for preventing and controlling potential cross-border disease outbreaks as a key component of the post-Ebola health systems recovery strategy and overall subregional health systems strengthening efforts.

An Integrated Surveillance and Response Network: The Investment Case

This section makes an investment case for the establishment of an integrated RDSR network in West Africa by exploring the qualitative evidence of the impact of regional networking on a country's disease surveillance and response systems, and provides guidance on the structure and functions of the network. It also serves to lay the analytical foundation for exploring options for financing and sustaining the cost of an RDSR network in the subregion and includes recommendations that can be applied to government-led efforts to increase health financing allocation for an effective and efficient early warning surveillance, preparedness, and response system required for building the resilience of health systems to infectious disease outbreaks.

Country Disease Surveillance and Response Systems: Key Findings

Assessments conducted in several countries in West Africa (including Guinea, Liberia, and Sierra Leone), preliminary results from the country profile exercise carried out by the World Health Organization (WHO),[4] and the lessons learned from EVD outbreaks reveal some key weaknesses of country health systems for infectious disease surveillance, preparedness, and response. The main findings that emerge from these assessments, and are identified as common weaknesses that have a negative impact on the effectiveness of DSR systems across countries in the subregion (including Guinea, Liberia, and Sierra Leone), include the following issues:

- A "fit-for-purpose" health workforce for disease surveillance, preparedness, and response is lacking at each level of the health system.

- A community-level surveillance, preparedness, and response structure does not exist or needs significant improvement.

- The laboratory infrastructure that is needed for timely and quality diagnosis of epidemic-prone diseases is limited.

- The lack of interoperability of different information systems hampers the analysis and utilization of information for decision making and actions that are required for disease mitigation measures.

- Infection prevention and control standards, infrastructure, and practices are inadequate.

- The management of the supply chain system that is crucial for coordinating surveillance, preparedness, and response activities is inefficient.

- There are major gaps in surge capacity for outbreak response, stockpiling of essential goods, information sharing, and collaboration.

Similar findings are also documented in the Global Health Security Agenda baseline assessments in a number of countries, including Guinea, Liberia, and Sierra Leone.

These findings highlight the need to adopt more effective mechanisms that enhance country health systems and promote regional collaboration in dealing with infectious disease outbreak threats in high-risk countries and in rapidly containing the spread to other neighboring countries in the subregion. Such a response must be built up in the broader context of developing effective institutions to perform core public health functions on a routine basis.

Overview of the Methodology

A qualitative case study methodology is adopted to answer the research question "What is the evidence for the value-added benefits of investing in an integrated, cross-sectoral regional disease surveillance and response network?"

Using a temporal comparison approach, the status of disease surveillance and response in regions with a well-established RDSR network, and its impact on the health system of member countries belonging to the network, is assessed. As applicable, an analysis of the counterfactual scenario—the absence of a regional network in the region under study—is also provided. In recognizing that there is no clear measure of the effectiveness or cost-effectiveness of infectious disease surveillance and response systems, an attempt to provide a qualitative assessment of the empirical evidence of the benefit of investing in an RDSR network and the impact on the overall health sector uses indicators categorized under four key pillars: (1) epidemiologic measures, (2) indicators assessing improved compliance with IHR (2005) via the development of country core capacities, (3) health systems strengthening indicators, and (4) measures of multisectoral and regional cooperation.

Overall, the analysis of the value added by investing in regional networking is based on the theoretical probability that such a network will lead to the implementation of more effective prevention measures and better containment of outbreak threats of epidemic potential, both nationally and regionally. It does this by complementing and enhancing existing systems and interventions put in place by country governments and other development partners to strengthen the national disease surveillance, preparedness, and response capacities of individual countries.

Case Studies of Successful Surveillance and Response Networks

Successful regional programs for the control of infectious diseases, both within and outside the region, have demonstrated the effectiveness and efficiency of a regionally coordinated approach to disease surveillance, preparedness, and response. Identified networks adopted as case studies include (1) the Pacific Public Health Surveillance Network (PPHSN); (2) the Mekong Basin Disease Surveillance (MBDS) network; (3) the East Africa Infectious Disease Surveillance Network (EAIDSNet); (4) the Middle East Consortium for Infectious Disease Surveillance (MECIDS) network; and (5) the Southern Africa Consortium for Infectious Disease Surveillance (SACIDS) network. The regions with existing networks were selected based on the quality of their past and recent responses to emerging and reemerging infectious disease outbreaks of public health significance, including avian and human influenza, EVD, dengue fever, severe acute respiratory syndrome (SARS), and West Nile virus.

Key findings from the analysis can be summarized as follows:

1. **Pacific Public Health Surveillance Network (PPHSN).** Established in the Pacific Island region in 1996, the PPSHN was instrumental in providing early warnings of emerging and reemerging infectious diseases of epidemic potential. It also served as the building block for the prioritization of streamlined reporting of regional surveillance of disease outbreaks (such as SARS, Dengue fever, measles, and influenza) that pose a threat to global health security across 22 Pacific Island countries.

2. **Mekong Basin Disease Surveillance (MBDS) network.** Founded in 1999, networking activities under the MBDS network improved the core capacity of member countries in areas such as cross-border surveillance and health workforce training in epidemiology, disease surveillance, preparedness, and response. The MBDS network has also resulted in strengthened multisectoral collaboration on surveillance and response and the establishment of multisectoral border response teams (MBRTs), which consist of trained officials representing the health, animal, customs, and immigration sector. Outbreaks averted in member countries that can be attributed to the presence of the MBDS network in the region include avian influenza, dengue fever, and typhoid fever.

3. **East Africa Infectious Disease Surveillance Network (EAIDSNet).** Since its formation in 2001, the EAIDSNet in the East Africa region has improved the surveillance and preparedness capacity of member countries of the East Africa Community (Burundi, Kenya, Rwanda, Tanzania, and Uganda) to respond to threats posed by infectious diseases in the region, using a OneHealth approach to strengthen the region's cross-border animal and human disease prevention and control efforts. Networking activities under the EAIDSNet also led to the early detection and effective control of four EVD outbreaks with high epidemic potential in Uganda and neighboring countries between 2000 and 2012. It was effective because it improved the countries' core public health capacities, which consequently led to quicker detection and decreased time to respond to disease outbreaks of international concern.

4. **Middle East Consortium for Infectious Disease Surveillance (MECIDS) network.** Established in 2003, the MECIDS network has resulted in effective collaboration across member countries in areas including the harmonization of diagnostic and reporting methodologies, common training for the health workforce in core skillsets, and increased cross-border collaboration for dealing with avian influenza outbreaks. Over the years, the three countries in the MECIDS network have demonstrated improved IHR core capacities in preparing and responding to new outbreaks, including prompt and coordinated border and airport screening, laboratory testing, common communication strategy, transparent reporting, and information exchange.

5. **Southern Africa Consortium for Infectious Disease Surveillance (SACIDS) Network.** Established in 2009, the SACIDS network has contributed toward building academic training and research capacity development across countries in the Southern Africa region and the effective use of information and communication technology (ICT) to improve risk communication on infectious disease outbreak threats.

Table C.2 in appendix C provides a full list of indicators and main findings from the analysis.

Critical Elements of an Effective and Efficient Surveillance and Response Network

Based on the analysis, four key elements have been identified as essential to the full functionality and efficiency of a cross-sectoral RDSR network in West Africa. Under each component, activities have been identified that contribute toward both building the core capacities of countries under the IHR (2005) and promoting regional cooperation among countries in the subregion in disease surveillance, preparedness, and response (see table C.3 in appendix C). It is vital that all three countries take these four elements into account in their plans and costing:

1. **Surveillance and Early Reporting Systems.** These are surveillance information systems that ensure the interoperability of country disease surveillance systems across the different tiers of the health system (community, local/district, and national levels) and across the animal and human health sector; they use early reporting and surveillance data to implement early prevention and control interventions.

2. **Laboratory Strengthening.** Improving laboratory functions for surveillance and response will require the identification of well-equipped and effective regional laboratory networks that contribute toward strengthening the capacities of national veterinary and public health laboratories and institutes, especially in the areas of case confirmation (including the facilitation of specimen transportation between national and regional reference laboratories), pathology, and the monitoring of trends in antimicrobial and insecticide resistance.

3. **Improved Preparedness and Rapid Response.** Improving the capacity of the health system to be better prepared to minimize the risks posed by infectious disease outbreaks calls for the establishment of a cross-sectoral, regional coordination structure that will function as a learning arm to share best practices and lessons learned across countries in the region. It can also serve as a central stockpiling unit to improve supply chain logistics management and planning for West African countries.

4. **Enhancing HRH Capacity and the Retention of a Skilled Health Workforce.** This requires addressing core HRH needs, including the training and retention of epidemiologists, laboratory personnel, entomologists, and ICT experts; and support for the identification and training of a multidisciplinary rapid response teams. A thorough health workforce mapping and planning initiative is needed across countries in the region to address the low retention rates of trained workers; to improve recruitment practices of skilled personnel; to support the development of roadmaps required for the institutionalization of identified pools of experts; and to address long-term health workforce needs in the region.

Investing in an RDSR network is a proactive, cost-effective approach that contributes toward the development of country core capacities under the International Health Regulations (IHR) adopted in 2005, and has the potential to reduce pandemic response fatigue that commonly occurs after the initial emergency response window is over. Furthermore, it can reduce the cost of contagion avoidance resulting from infectious disease outbreaks. A well-coordinated, cross-sectoral approach to transnational disease surveillance and response in West Africa can also increase the value of ongoing and future disease control and prevention efforts in the region by (1) catalyzing the development of innovative platforms and approaches adopted to reduce mortality and morbidity due to infectious diseases; (2) encouraging improved data sharing and coordination across various sectors as well as interoperability of disease surveillance and reporting across the different tiers of the health system; (3) encouraging novel methods of understanding infectious disease dynamics; and (4) strengthening existing partnerships and developing new partnerships at the country, regional, and global levels.

Operational and Fixed Costs for a Surveillance and Response Network

An estimation of the operational and fixed costs needed to establish and maintain an RDSR network is necessary to determine funding gaps, to calculate the return on investments, and to plan better for the identification of resources to ensure its long-term sustainability. The IHR (2005) monitoring framework provides a platform to estimate one-time capital costs and annual recurrent costs based on preidentified variables such as population size, existing infrastructure, and the population's health status (Katz et al. 2012). Part of the analysis explored the use of the IHR monitoring framework to estimate the fixed and operating costs of implementing the eight core capacities of the IHR (2005), including the cost of activities identified under each core capacity. The annual cost of meeting the requirements set out in the IHR (2005) and the equivalent Organization for Animal Health (OIE) standards in 139 developing countries is estimated to be US$3.4 billion (World Bank 2012). It is estimated that more than 50 percent of these costs would be operating costs and the other half would be investments in hardware (laboratories, equipment) and human resources capacity building. For a model Southeast Asian country X scenario, the total annual fixed and operating cost for meeting these requirements is estimated at between approximately US$231 million and US$283 million (table 4.1) This estimate is based on a population size of 60 million, 64 provinces, 600 functional districts, and 6 officially designated points of entry; and 1 ministry of health responsible for public health surveillance, response, and laboratory capacities at the national, provincial, district, and community levels).

TABLE 4.1

The Estimated Annual Costs of International Health Regulations Core Capacities, 2005

U.S. dollars

Core capacity	Fixed cost	Operating cost
National legislation, policy, and financing	75,000	0
Coordination and national focal points communication	823,102	347,959– 88,868
Surveillance	5,261,764	26,238,293–69,606,113
Response	20,480,332	3,981,294–5,215,857
Preparedness	2,889,166	103,726,507–103,786,408
Risk communications	4,389	1,868,869– 2,141,939
Human resources	4,389	620,649–653,009
Laboratories	49,619,443	13,742,692–20,057,218
Points of entry[a]	153,062	838,851–1,435,767
Total	79,310,647	151,365,114–203,485,179
Total cost: Fixed and operating		230,675,761–282,795,826

Source: Katz et al. 2012.

Note: The cost estimate for each component is based on a model Southeast Asian country (country X) with a population of 60 million; 64 provinces, 600 functional districts, and 6 officially designated points of entry; and 1 ministry of health responsible for public health surveillance, response, and laboratory capacities at the national, provincial, district, and community levels. The cost estimate excludes the cost of surveillance and response within the veterinary health system. The annual cost of the requirement for meeting the IHR (2005) and equivalent OIE standards in 139 developing countries is estimated at US$3.4 billion (World Bank 2012).

a. Although *points of entry* is not a core capacity, it is an area of weakness that needs to be strengthened to minimize public health risks caused by the spread of diseases via international traffic.

Taking a closer look at data on a cross-sectoral, disease-specific surveillance system, the World Bank reviewed data from 46 countries to estimate total incremental budget needs to bring country surveillance systems up to OIE and WHO standards for the prevention and control of avian influenza (table 4.2; World Bank 2012).[5] The study concluded that 45 percent of the total incremental budget was allocated to animal health, 41 percent to human health, and 14 percent to joint planning and communication activities. Furthermore, 55 percent was allocated to recurrent costs and 45 percent to investment costs. Among the 23 countries in Sub-Saharan Africa for which data were available, the animal health services require, on average, US$1.2 million per country per year (around US$0.14 per head of poultry per year).[6] In the same sample of countries,

TABLE 4.2

Estimated Annual Costs to Bring Surveillance and Response Systems up to OIE/WHO Standards: Fixed and Operating Costs, West African Countries

U.S. dollars

Core capacity	Fixed cost (US$)	Operating cost (US$)	Total	Percent
National legislation, policy, and financing	92,393.14	n.a.	92,393.14	0.03
Coordination and national focal points communication	1,013,986.35	191,064.54	1,205,050.89	0.41
Surveillance	6,482,011.76	32,301,849.37	38,783,861.13	20.72
Response	25,229,894.95	3,128,681.90	28,358,576.84	9.77
Preparedness	3,559,188.14	69,857,973.67	73,417,161.81	41.54
Risk communications	5,406.85	1,373,276.41	1,378,683.25	0.78
Human resources	5,406.85	346,304.48	351,711.33	0.19
Laboratories	61,126,613.29	11,416,106.47	72,542,719.75	25.91
Points of entry[a]	188,558.38	800,082.78	988,641.15	0.50
Total	97,703,459.69	119,415,339.62	217,118,799.30	100%

Sources: Based on parameters from Global Health Risk and Financing Framework Commission 2016; and Katz et al. 2012.
Note: n.a. = not applicable; OIE = World Organizaiton for Animal Health; WHO = World Health Organization.
a. Although *points of entry* is not a core capacity, it is an area of weakness that needs to be strengthened to minimize public health risks caused by the spread of diseases via international traffic.

human health surveillance and response services required, on average, US$1.3 million per country per year (about US$0.10 per capita per year), with 36 percent allocated to prevention and 64 percent to control (World Bank 2012). Table 4.3 displays the cost requirements, disaggregated by type of service (prevention and control). The total annual cost is estimated at US$84.95 million, of which US$51.55 million is for animal health and US$33.4 million for human health.[7]

To calculate specific costs of operating an RDSR network tailored to the West African country context, further costing exercises will need to use existing public health surveillance costing platforms, such as the Integrated Disease Surveillance and Response (IDSR) SurvCost Tool developed by the U.S. Centers for Disease Control and Prevention.

The analysis given above takes into account the different variables that are essential investments required to implement the IHR (2005) core capacities and to bring surveillance and response systems up to the standards of the WHO and OIE (table 4.2). However, the proposed annual

TABLE 4.3

Estimated Costs to Bring Surveillance and Response Systems up to OIE/WHO Standards: Disaggregated by Type of Service, West African Countries

U.S. dollars

Animal health service	Investment	Recurrent	Human health service	Investment	Recurrent
Prevention			**Prevention**		
Surveillance	5,155,052	3,093,031	Surveillance	1,670,145	1,670,145
Laboratory diagnostic capacity	2,577,526	1,546,516	Laboratory diagnostic capacity	1,002,087	1,336,116
Biosecurity inspection	1,031,010	1,031,010			
Control			**Control**		
Quarantine, vaccination, hygiene programs	4,639,547	3,093,031	Rapid response and isolation	2,004,174	2,004,174
Culling	515,505	1,031,010	Vaccination and hygiene programs	4,342,376	2,004,174
Compensation	515,505	2,577,526			
Other costs		24,744,250	**Other costs**		17,369,504
Total costs		51,550,519	**Total costs**		33,402,895

Source: Based on parameters from World Bank 2012.
Note: OIE = World Organization for Animal Health; WHO = World Health Organization.

cost estimates provided in table 4.2 are not comparable with the cost estimates provided in the health services strengthening investment plans for Guinea, Liberia, and Sierra Leone for the following reasons: (1) the three countries have outlined specific investments in activities related to improving epidemic preparedness, surveillance, and response, at different capacities; (2) the individual country plans account for cross-cutting investments (that are not limited to disease surveillance and response), including the scaling up of HRH, strengthening national centers of excellence and training centers, and increasing access to HRH training programs. These activities are embedded under different pillars related to HRH and overall health systems strengthening; and (3) the analysis considers the cost of meeting the health workforce needs specifically as it relates to surveillance, preparedness, and response. Assessing the HRH needs for epidemic preparedness, surveillance, and response will require a thorough needs assessment, followed by a costing exercise and gap analysis tailored to the individual country context.

Tables C.4 and C.5 in appendix C provide a summary of the priority pillars outlined in the plans for improving surveillance, preparedness, and response in Guinea, Liberia, and Sierra Leone, and the estimated costs associated with these pillars.

Factors to Ensure the Sustainability of Financing a Surveillance and Response Network

The sustainability of a regional network in the long term requires a high level of government prioritization as well as intergovernmental and regional cooperation in providing an RDSR network as a global public good. Globally, the occurrence of new infectious disease outbreaks is becoming a common trend. Analysis of temporal trends in global disease outbreaks that occurred between 1980 and 2010 shows an increase in the total number of outbreaks and the complexities in the detection and response to the causal diseases, of which

FIGURE 4.1

Global Number of Human Infectious Disease Outbreaks and Complexity of Causal Diseases, 1980–2010

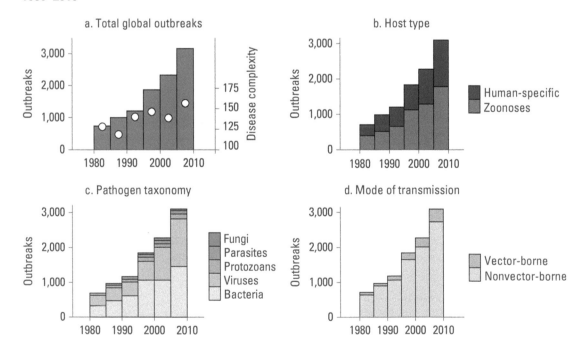

Source: Smith et al. 2014. Reprinted with permission.
Note: In panel a, the bars represent total global outbreaks, and the dots represent the total number of diseases causing outbreaks in each year.

FIGURE 4.2

Number of Infectious Disease Outbreaks per Year Reported by the WHO, Global Estimates

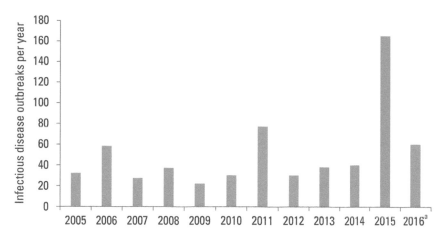

Note: WHO = World Health Organization.

a. The 2016 bar shows data for the first three months of 2016 only.

approximately 60 percent were caused by infectious diseases of animal origins, including H5N1, EVD, severe acute respiratory syndrome (SARS), human immunodeficiency virus (HIV), and Middle East respiratory syndrome (figure 4.1). In 2015 alone, approximately 165 infectious disease outbreaks of epidemic potential were officially reported by the WHO, an estimate representing a 5.5-fold increase over the frequency of outbreaks reported in 2010 (figure 4.2). Consequently, as infectious disease outbreak threats grow, the probability of the occurrence of a pandemic also becomes higher, with the expected annual economic loss due to a pandemic estimated at US$60 billion (GHRF Commission 2016).[8]

As evidenced by the increasing frequency of emerging and reemerging infectious disease outbreaks—including EVD, highly pathogenic avian influenza (HPAI H5N1),[9] and the Zika virus—a health threat in any country can develop into a health threat everywhere, and an uncontrolled outbreak at its source is very likely to easily spread to other countries via increased travel, trade, and interaction between humans and livestock (see figure 4.3) (Kilpatrick and Randolph 2012). Given the transboundary nature of infectious diseases, and because a significant number (more than 60 percent) of disease pathogens can be transmitted between animals and humans, the need is critical for better coordination and exchange of knowledge and information among countries, and between the animal health and human health sectors.

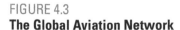

FIGURE 4.3
The Global Aviation Network

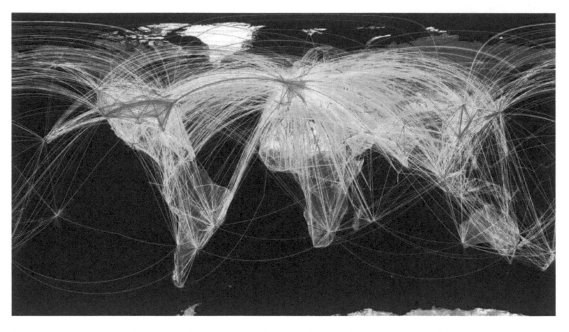

Source: Reprinted from *The Lancet,* 380, A. Marm Kilpatrick and Sarah E. Randolph, "Zoonoses 2: Drivers, Dynamics, and Control of Emerging Zoonotic Diseases." 1946–55 (2012), Elsevier. Used with permission. Additional permission required for re-use.
Note: The network depicts the transboundary nature of infectious disease outbreaks. The lines show direct links between airports. Passenger capacity is indicated by the color of the lines: red = thousands of people per day; yellow = hundreds; blue = tens.

Routes linking regions at similar latitudes (in the Northern or Southern hemispheres) represent pathways that pathogens can move along to reach novel regions.

An investment in an RDSR network in West Africa will serve to enhance public health and veterinary health systems required to tackle infectious diseases threats, including the burden of endemic diseases, and will contribute toward improving the effectiveness of disease control programs of countries in the subregion. Mainstreaming networking activities into health systems strengthening activities of countries in the subregion is crucial to fully develop and sustain the network's institutional capacity to prevent or control the spread of infectious disease outbreaks before they can become large-scale epidemics. Such investment must be made within the broader context of developing effective institutions to perform core public health functions on a routine basis. Given the volatility of donor funding, innovative financing tools and funding mechanisms that provide new ways to create long-term, predictable funding streams need to be explored. Based on an initial review of the literature (International Office of Migration 2009), the following possible financing options have been identified:

- Long-term twinning arrangements between human and animal health institutes of high-income and resource-poor countries, funded by specific budget lines in high-income countries

- The establishment of a global financing framework for the implementation of the IHR (2005) / IDSR strategy with each individual country's contribution proportional to its national income

- The introduction of social impact bonds under a corporate social responsibility financing agreement, as a framework for investing in systems for the prevention of infectious disease outbreaks

- Micro levies on cooperation (such as the aviation and transportation industries) as part of cross-sectoral cooperation in disease surveillance and response

- Climate change financing

- Solidarity levies

- The establishment of special endowments through nonconventional donors

- The imposition of a levy on internationally traded meat

- Public-private partnerships for the provision of certain activities under an RDSR network

Based on the alternative financing options identified (see also table C.5 in appendix C for external financing options), medium- and long-term financing scenarios will need to be estimated and linked to current and expected trends in total government health expenditures and to development assistance to health as well as other macroeconomic indicators, such as external trade and economic growth.

Conclusions

This chapter adopted a collective case study methodology to assess the benefit of investing in an integrated RDSR network and its impact on health systems strengthening efforts, especially in the context of Guinea, Liberia, and Sierra Leone. Some success stories both within and outside the Sub-Saharan Africa region have shown the benefit of regional networking arrangements for overall health systems strengthening for effective surveillance, preparedness, and response. In the case of Uganda, the country's membership in the EAIDSNet led to the early detection and effective control of multiple Ebola outbreaks with high epidemic potential that occurred between 2000 and 2012 through the successful establishment of Village Health Teams and the introduction of the District Health Information System, as part of network activities for effective surveillance and response (Ope et al. 2013). Recognized as the site of the largest outbreak of EVD prior to the devastating outbreak of 2014 in West Africa, Uganda has shown great leadership in controlling the spread of EVD and curtailing the spread of the virus to neighboring countries by improving its core public health capacities over the years, as mandated under the IHR (2005).

Overall, the health systems of countries within the East African Community have benefited immensely from their individual country's membership in the EAIDSNet. Regional network activities have resulted in the institutionalization of a formal health department within the East African Community to address broader health challenges in the region that encompass surveillance—including maternal and neonatal child health systems strengthening, research and development, and food safety and regulations. Other successes include the development of preparedness and response capacities of member countries under the PPHSN, MBDS, MECIDS, and SACIDS Network.

Given the rise in the total number of outbreaks of epidemic potential and the transboundary nature of infectious diseases, including those of animal origin, the analysis considers the different variables that are essential investments required to implement the IHR (2005) core capacities of countries and to bring surveillance and response systems up to the standards of the WHO and the OIE. Findings from the analysis and the successes highlighted in this chapter emphasize the importance and the need for country governments and development partners to prioritize investments in cross-border and cross-sectoral initiatives for strengthening country disease surveillance and response systems, including financing the establishment of a sustainable RDSR network in West Africa. Such a cross-border and cross-sectoral approach to epidemic preparedness, surveillance, and response is currently not addressed under the investment plans of Guinea, Liberia, and Sierra Leone. Investments in an RDSR network in West Africa will serve to strengthen the capacity of national public health and veterinary health systems to provide early warnings of infectious disease outbreak threats; improve epidemic preparedness and response capacities; and, in the medium to long terms, will yield a high economic return on investments for member countries and the subregion.

Notes

1. The WHO International Health Regulations (IHR 2005) requires country governments to develop, strengthen, and maintain the core capacities of national public health systems to detect, assess, notify, and respond promptly and effectively to health risks and public health emergencies of international concern. A revised version of the IHR 2005 came into force on June 15, 2007 (see http://www.who.int/ihr/publications/9789241596664/en/) aiming to "prevent, protect against, control and provide a public health response to the international spread of disease in ways that are commensurate with and restricted to public health risks, and which avoid unnecessary interference with international traffic and trade."

2. The eight core capacities required for the implementation of the IHR (2005) at the country level are national legislation, policy and financing; coordination and national focal point communication; surveillance; preparedness; response; risk communication; human resources; and laboratories. additionally, points of entry is identified as an area of weakness that needs to be strengthened in order to minimize public health risks caused by the spread of diseases via international traffic.

3. These figures are derived from the results of the economic analysis of the Regional Disease Surveillance Systems Enhancement (REDISSE) project, and are based on the observation of past influenza pandemics that occurred in the 20th century.

4. In January 2016, the WHO commenced a country profile exercise, on behalf of the World Bank, in several countries in West Africa, including Guinea, Liberia, and Sierra Leone. The objective of the exercise is to provide an overview of the status of disease surveillance and response (DSR) systems of countries and to provide recommendations for building surveillance, preparedness, and response capacities of countries as a critical step toward investing in an RDSR network (see table C.1 in appendix C for the scope of the country profile exercise).

5. The 46 countries in this study were mostly in Sub-Saharan Africa, and also included a few countries in Southern Asia, Latin America, Europe, and the Middle East.

6. 1 poultry = 0.015 Livestock Units (LSU) (World Bank and TAFS 2011).

7. West Africa's population in 2013 = 334,028,922. Head of poultry (that is, all poultry, including chicken, ducks, and geese) in 2005 = 368,218,000 (1 head of poultry = 0.015 LSU); World Bank Development Indicators 2016 and FAO 2007, respectively.

8. The total annual benefit of avoiding a pandemic in West Africa is, on average, equal to US$7.2 billion.

9. H5N1 was declared an epidemic in January 2015 in Nigeria, followed by Burkina Faso, Niger, Ghana, and Côte d'Ivoire. A previous H5N1 outbreak had occurred between 2006 and 2009 in the region; that outbreak triggered an international response that contributed to eradicating the disease.

References

GHRF Commission (Global Health Risk Framework for the Future Commission). 2016. *The Neglected Dimension of Global Security: A Framework to Counter Infectious Disease Crises.* Washington, DC: National Academies Press.

Katz, Rebecca, Vibhuti Haté, Sarah Kornblet, and Julie E. Fischer. 2012. "Costing Framework for International Health Regulations (2005)." *Emerging Infectious Diseases* 18 (7): 1121–27.

Kilpatrick, A. Marm, and Sarah E. Randolph. 2012. "Zoonoses 2: Drivers, Dynamics, and Control of Emerging Zoonotic Diseases." *The Lancet* 380 (1–7 December): 1946–55.

Ope, Maurice, Stanley Sonoiya, James Kariuki, Leonard Mboera, Gandham Ramana, Miriam Schneidman, and Mwihaki Kimura. 2013. "Regional Initiatives in Support of Surveillance East Africa: The East Africa Integrated Disease Surveillance Network (EAIDSNet) Experience." *Emerging Health Threats Journal* 6. https://www.ncbi.nlm .nih.gov/pmc/articles/PMC3557906/.

Smith, Katherine F., Michael Goldberg, Samantha Rosenthal, Lynn Carlson, Jane Chen, Cici Chen, and Sohini Ramachandran. 2014. "Global Rise in Human Infectious Disease Outbreaks." *Journal of the Royal Society Interface* 11: 2014.0950.

UNDG (United Nations Development Group). 2015. *Socio-Economic Impact of Ebola Virus Disease in West African Countries: A Call for National and Regional Containment, Recovery and Prevention.* United Nations Development Group, Western and Central Africa. http://www.africa.undp.org /content/dam/rba/docs/Reports/ebola-west-africa.pdf.

World Bank. 2012. *People Pathogens and Our Planet: The Economics of One Health.* Washington, DC: World Bank.

CHAPTER 5

Overall Conclusions and Recommendations

Introduction

This book set out to identify the requirements for strengthening the health systems of Guinea, Liberia, and Sierra Leone—comparing it to proposals in the national investment plans of these countries—in order to lay the foundation for sound public health policies and establish regional disease surveillance networks. As noted, the aim of this book is to go beyond merely bringing the number of Ebola cases to zero in these countries, but instead to help them build viable, realistic, and sustainable health systems so that they can realize their aspirations of achieving universal health coverage and can anticipate and deal with epidemics. It is hoped that such a roadmap would also be of benefit to other developing countries that either confront similar situations or may do so in the future. The main conclusions and recommendations are summarized below.

Health System Strengthening Plans and Fiscal Space

This study has reviewed the costed national investment plans prepared by the three governments and analyzed their viability, realism, and implications. It has explored options for expanding the fiscal space for health. This section presents key recommendations for the countries as a group, adds specific additional items for individual counties (where appropriate), identifies good practice examples, and lays out actions that the World Bank might take to support health system strengthening.

Recommendations for All Three Countries

Engage in an inclusive universal health coverage (UHC) process as soon as possible. The two biggest challenges at this level are: (1) the implementation of a plan to cover the poorest and most vulnerable through public funds and (2) the introduction of collective and strategic thinking about the possibility of including in the plan coverage of the informal sector. To achieve this, each of the three governments should (1) undertake a study on the exact situation of health financing, (2) define a health financing strategy and universal coverage policy, (3) develop a law that provides the legal basis for UHC, (4) start the progressive implementation of UHC policy, and (5) prepare the necessary implementing legislation and put in place the institutions and tools for the first steps of UHC.

To boost the performance of the health sector in the three countries, it is necessary to move from inputs-based financing systems to performance-based financing (PBF) systems. In Sierra Leone, the current PBF program should be improved. In Guinea and Liberia, it becomes essential to think of developing and implementing a PBF strategy (starting with a pilot) where the efforts, resources, and attention are focused on results rather than inputs.

Harmonize the planning, medium-term budgeting, and annual budgeting processes. Like most developing countries, the dichotomy between planning (development of health plans), Medium-Term Expenditure Frameworks (MTEF), and annual budgets in Guinea, Liberia, and Sierra Leone do not allow for an appropriate translation of planned activities into codified budget lines. For that reason, these plans and MTEFs are likely to remain theoretical exercises unless ministries of health work closely with key central departments, such as finance and planning, and with other relevant sectoral ministries to harmonize the plans and translate them into working documents. The introduction of a multiyear programmatic budgeting with a flexible and simplified budget line classification would, for example, be a major asset in improving the evidence-based planning and budgeting of all public sectors, including health.

This exercise of harmonization must be accompanied by a results-based approach. The public financial management (PFM), the public auditing, and the control processes must be improved for all sectors, including health. However, the public control process should also include monitoring results. To do this requires a results-based budgeting where multiyear budgets include not only labels/items and amounts, but also results/indicators in front of budget paragraphs. The Ministry of Health and other public departments should be judged more in relation to the completion of these results than in relation to the execution of such rigid and extremely complex budgets.

Guinea should increase the priority of the health sector in its budget. The Guinean government allocates only 4 percent of its budget to the health sector, as compared to 15 percent in Liberia, 11 percent in Sierra Leone, and an average of 10 percent in Sub-Saharan Africa. With this low prioritization, the health sector cannot be strengthened, and consequently will stay fragile and vulnerable to all threats and epidemics. That is why it is necessary to expand the fiscal space for health Guinea through, among others avenues, a more substantial budget allocation. It is improbable that Guinea will reach the Abuja Declaration rate of 15 percent in the short or medium terms for practical reasons pertaining to public finance constraints and absorption capacity. But in the long term, the government could increase its health budget by 2 percent over a period of three to four years to reach the Sub-Saharan African average of 10 percent.

The Role of the World Bank

The World Bank has a comparative advantage and capacity in terms of high technical assistance in the area of health financing, results-based financing, and evidence-based planning and budgeting. Three areas in which the World Bank may be of assistance are as follows:

Technical assistance in evidence-based planning and budgeting and the development of health financing and UHC strategies: Planning and budgeting should be strengthened through a mix of capacity building (through, for example, study tours, training, and technical assistance for analysis) and analysis of information (for example, public expenditure review, fiscal space analyses, and national health accounts). Through the Global Financing Facility for Every Woman and Every Child (GFF) process, the governments and their partners can undertake an inclusive process for preparing a comprehensive, coherent, efficient, and realistic health financing strategy and UHC policy.

Results-oriented lending: Performance-based financing strategies—or their improvement, in the case of Sierra Leone—would increase provider and, possibly, user incentives for health provision and use. This could be done through a mix of performance-based financing (providers) and conditional (or unconditional) cash transfers for users. Strengthening the accountability and incentives for results should increase the systems' performance and efficiency.

The World Bank's convening power: The World Bank should use its convening power to ensure that the recommendations of this study find the necessary traction. Following the Geneva high-level meeting, this report and country progress reports on their plans should be presented at an international conference to validate the conclusions and jointly define next steps, roles and responsibilities, and monitoring mechanisms.

Human Resources for Health

In all three countries, the need to strengthen the number and distribution of sufficiently skilled and competent human resources at all levels of the health system is critical, and the objective and specific interventions are outlined in the countries' investment plans. Although important elements needed to increase the stock, distribution, and performance of human resources for health (HRH) are included in all three investment plans, the implementation of these plans will require a particular strong focus on training the right health workers for the right locations: that is, a fit-for-purpose health workforce that is appropriate and responsive to the needs of each country.

Chapter 3 provides a closer insight into the health worker scaling-up ambitions of the three countries as well as the implications of reaching set scaling-up targets on meeting needs and fiscal space realities. The report finds that reaching the health worker scaling-up targets identified in the investment plans (and the accompanying costing exercises) will not substantially improve health worker densities (when taking into account projected population growth), particularly in Guinea and Sierra Leone. Furthermore, although projected fiscal space in all three countries is likely to be sufficient to reach investment plan scaling-up targets (as well as international thresholds of 2.5 doctors, nurses, and midwives per 1,000 population), it is insufficient when taking into account all other health worker cadres on the public payroll. Ambitions to reach target densities and international thresholds would significantly stretch already-limited production capacity for nurses, midwives, and doctors. And, finally, a predominant focus on scaling up higher-level cadres in urban training environments will do little to address rural/urban imbalances of health workers.

Recommendations for All Three Countries

To address prevailing needs within a constrained fiscal space scenario, a paradigm shift as to *who* to train and *how* to train health workers is needed in all three countries. The immediate focus in all three countries needs to be on scaling up their rural health workforce. The biggest challenge in all countries is not the lack of health workers available at the aggregate level, but the shortage of those available in rural areas. The investment plans' emphasis on the scaling up of (urban-trained) mid- and higher-level cadres may worsen the rural/urban maldistribution of health workers. While high-level cadres and urban training environments play an important role in each of these countries, in particular in meeting faculty needs, secondary- and tertiary-level service delivery needs, and private sector demand, public sector investments should prioritize the production of health workers with the greatest social rates of return, focusing on competencies needed for UHC, and ensuring their presence in parts of the country where needs are greatest.

The emphasis needs to be on innovative training policies, in particular rural pipeline policies, to scale up the health workforce in rural areas. When *combined* with country- and cadre-specific monetary and non-monetary incentive policies, such policies hold the potential for addressing many of the concerns related to HRH in all three countries. The specifics of such policies will vary from country to country and from health worker to health worker. *Rural pipeline policies* refer to decentralized training approaches where health workers *from* rural areas are trained *in* rural areas and *for* rural areas, and provided the continuous support, supervision, and mentorship needed to ensure their retention. The logic is that health workers who are familiar with rural surroundings and who are tied to their friends and families are much more likely to work in such environments upon graduation than their urban counterparts.

Such strategies should be combined with a focus on scaling up lower-level and mid-level cadres; this is not only more cost-effective, but it is also linked to increased rural employment uptake and retention. Lower-level cadres such as auxiliary cadres, health assistants, and technologists tend to be more willing to work in rural areas than higher- and mid-level cadres. Furthermore, the production of cadres specific to rural and remote areas (and thus less competitive in the national and international level market) is a promising strategy, often combined with a rural pipeline approach.

The emphasis on community health worker (CHW) scaling up in all three countries is notable, but should be carefully considered and not seen as an end in itself. The extent to which CHWs are integrated within a broader frontline health worker team and system, horizontally trained and supervised and accepted by their peers and their community, is a critical aspect of their potential success. Plans for community health volunteer (CHV) and CHW developments should be integrated into broader health workforce planning; such plans require further evidence-based analysis and policy dialogue to ensure that the programs take a labor market perspective and represent the most efficient investment in workforce development to achieve health goals.

Innovative training approaches for rural scaling up should be combined with a continued focus on ensuring and improving health worker performance. Numbers alone do not guarantee effective and sufficient service delivery outcomes, and health workers—particularly in rural areas—often exhibit low performance standards. Health worker performance should be understood to be a function of both capacity (supplies, knowledge) and effort (motivation), and weaknesses and solutions should be identified for each. On the knowledge front, assessments should be carried out to help identify constraint and strengthen competencies needed to achieve UHC, including on disease surveillance and response, for health workers across the health system.

While efforts to train an appropriate skill mix for UHC will yield improvements over the medium to long terms, this should be coupled with short-term capacity-building measures for existing health workers at all levels of the health system. Such measures are already in place in some countries and may require scaling up. Standardized, team-based short-term training programs and approaches, strengthened mentoring and opportunities for continuous professional development, and effective supportive supervision coupled with clearly defined referral structures and professional scopes of practice are all critical for success. In addition, such strategies should also be reinforced with appropriate, monetary and nonmonetary incentives, when these are based on evidence from health labor market assessments.

For all three countries, the specific interventions required to implement the investment plans will have to be informed by solid health education and labor market assessments. The mention of the importance of such studies in the investment plans of all three countries, in particular health labor market assessments, is a step in the right direction on this issue and needs to be supported by the World Bank immediately. This can be followed by collaborative efforts between the World Bank's Health and Education Department, as well as with key partners, including the WHO, to consider relevant, strategically practical investments.

The Role of the World Bank

The World Bank, in close collaboration with partners such as the WHO, is well equipped to provide the required support to each of the three countries on HRH. Analytical work needs to be followed by concerted investments geared toward developing and implementing innovative workforce solutions to support each country's move toward the development of a fit-for-purpose health workforce that is in line with the goals of greater resilience, efficiency, and UHC. The World Bank's comparative advantage in the area of health labor market analysis and support, together with its convening and lending power, renders the organization well placed to play a leading role on HRH in the three countries and in the region as a whole. Cross-sectoral collaboration within the World Bank and at the country level—in particular between the health, labor, and education sectors—will be critical to the success of any support.

Disease Surveillance

Recognizing the health system weaknesses that exist across countries in West Africa—including Guinea, Liberia, and Sierra Leone—there is heightened momentum to improve collaboration among countries in the subregion for the prevention and control of potential cross-border disease outbreaks, including those of zoonotic origins. The establishment of a regional disease surveillance and response (RDSR) network in West Africa serves as a critical step in the right direction that is well aligned with the region's ongoing political agenda of improving regional cooperation among countries. It is a key priority needed to make the necessary paradigm shift from the reactive approach usually adopted for the prevention, control, and response to infectious disease outbreaks in the region to a more preemptive and proactive risk reduction approach. However, an RDSR system is only as strong as its weakest link, given that a weakness in a member country's capacity for early detection, preparedness, and response to infectious disease outbreaks poses a threat to other countries belonging to the network and to overall global security. This, therefore, makes it imperative to enhance health systems by developing the core capacities identified under the *International Health Regulations (2005)*, 3rd ed. (WHO 2016) in order to establish an effective and efficient RDSR network that complements each country's disease surveillance and reporting systems and contributes toward strengthening country preparedness and response capacities. Such capacities must be built within the broader context of developing effective institutions to perform core public health functions on a routine basis.

Recommendations for All Three Countries

Invest in interoperable surveillance and early reporting systems and the interoperability of disease surveillance systems (across the different tiers of the health system) with other information systems across the human and animal health sectors. Enhance laboratory networking capacity for bio-surveillance and technical support for integrated laboratory information systems that are interoperable with disease surveillance and reporting systems.

Expand the HRH capacity for disease surveillance, emergency preparedness, and response, including the implementation of evidence-based policies to address regulatory issues that have an impact on the shortage and retention of a skilled health workforce. For each country, this will require thorough health workforce mapping and planning to assess and address the medium- to long-term health workforce needs of cadres across the different tiers of the health system; to improve recruitment practices of skilled personnel and address capacity building needs; and to support the development of roadmaps required for the institutionalization of identified pools of experts in disease surveillance and response (DSR).

Improve the preparedness and response capacity of countries and establish policies to promote cross-border and cross-sectoral collaboration in DSR systems. This includes strengthening early warning and response systems; updating and/or developing cross-sectoral emergency preparedness and response plans and ensuring their integration into the broader national all-hazards disaster risk management framework; and improving and harmonizing policies, legislation, and operating procedures for emergency response.

In terms of financing, overall findings from the analysis show that the establishment of an RDSR network is an economically sound investment that ensures better disaster risk management by enhancing the performance of health systems, via the development of the IHR (2005) core capacities, and promotes regional collaboration and coordination among countries in the subregion in the management of infectious disease outbreaks. The overall focus of such an investment is on strengthening the capacity of country health systems to manage infectious diseases threats, including those of animal origins, via a cross-sectoral approach that would be of ultimate benefit to both the human health and animal health sectors, and the entire region.

Investments in the establishment of an effective and efficient RDSR network in West Africa would serve to harness the power of other regional networks to improve regional and global cooperation by the Economic Community of West African States (ECOWAS) member countries for the attainment of better population health outcomes and to promote global health security. To ensure the sustainability of regional networking arrangements in disease surveillance and response, sustainable financing mechanisms need to be put in place by governments that will ultimately promote country ownership of the provision of an RDSR network in West Africa as a global public good.

Establishing a regional disease surveillance network (improving health systems capacity and service delivery platforms for effective surveillance and response) will require strengthening cross-sectoral capacity as well as regional cooperation to earlier detect, better prepare, and rapidly respond to infectious diseases threats at the animal-human-ecosystem interface. Key recommendations for achieving this goal are summarized as follows:

1. Make investments in human resources development skills mapping and planning that are critical for addressing the health workforce requirements for the full implementation of the IHR (2005) in ECOWAS member countries.

2. Adopt an integrated cross-sectoral approach to infectious disease surveillance and response at the country and regional levels to better understand the human-animal ecosystem interface given the increase in emerging and reemerging infectious diseases of animal origin, and establish interoperable surveillance and reporting systems across the different tiers of the health system.

3. Promote strong involvement of country and regional representatives in regular intercountry dialogues to share best practices and take stock of the state of disease surveillance and response in the region.

4. Establish links of an RDSR network with existing global notification systems—such as the WHO Global Outbreak Alert Response Network (GOARN), Event Management System (EMS), and Global Early Warning System (GLEWS)—and ensure the regular utilization of data for actions that prevent or control infectious diseases in the subregion.

5. Review and update existing action plans, such as Integrated National Action Plans (INAPs),[1] and prioritize investments for their implementation to improve the quality of animal and human public health systems to better respond to infectious disease threats.

6. Promote the transition of the Integrated Disease Surveillance and Response (IDSR) reporting platform from a paper-based system to an integrated electronic system of data collection and reporting backed up by a streamlined traditional paper-based system.

7. Ensure the linking of disease surveillance and response activities to environmental concerns such as climate change to ensure planning for the allocation of funds as part of government budget. This recommendation accounts for the importance of linking disease surveillance, preparedness, and response to the climate change agenda in recognition of the impact of climate change on disease outbreaks. It also acknowledges the importance of climate science tools to make early warning predictions and prevent climate-related health events.

8. Explore options for setting up an RDSR network as a foundation, which will represent a legal entity that is able to receive various sources of funding over the long term as part of efforts to promote long-term network sustainability.

The Role of the World Bank

The role of the World Bank in disease surveillance is threefold: its direct participation in the process through its financing of a new regional integration project; its expansion of cross-sectoral engagement in DSR across the animal, human, and environment sector to promote the operationalization of the OneHealth approach; and its essential role as a convener.

Participating in a new regional integration project. As part of the efforts to promote the regional cooperation and coordination required for enhancing the DSR capacity of country health systems, the World Bank is investing in a Regional Disease Surveillance Systems Enhancement (REDISSE) project that aims to strengthen cross-sectoral and regional capacity for integrated disease surveillance and response in West Africa. REDISSE is being prepared as a series of interdependent projects, an approach that provides a platform for high-level policy and regulatory harmonization, cooperation, and coordination among countries aiming to achieving benefits that will go beyond each country's boundaries. The estimated project financing for the first series of projects (SOP1) is US$230 million in country and regional International Development Association (IDA) funds. Countries included in SOP1 are Guinea, Liberia, and Sierra Leone, which bore the greatest burden of the EVD outbreak and are thus extremely vulnerable countries, as well as Nigeria and Senegal, which have more effective surveillance systems and serve as hosts for important regional assets.

Providing technical assistance to support the operationalization of OneHealth. REDISSE is under development jointly by the Health, Nutrition, and Population and the Agriculture Global practices of the World Bank to ensure that the human-animal interface is addressed as a practical step toward the implementation of the OneHealth approach. During the first year of project implementation in SOP1 countries, the World Bank will solicit the engagement of the environment sector both internally and externally. It will include analytical and operational research to obtain better clarity on the priorities for addressing the environmental interface of OneHealth and to identify the best options for expanding investments in the next series of projects.

Acting as convener. The World Bank is using its convening power to build a coalition of technical and financial partners engaged in disease surveillance, preparedness, and response, and to establish the momentum required to prioritize disease surveillance and response high on the agenda of country governments. A key priority will also involve strengthening the World Bank's engagement across the health, agriculture, and environment sectors to operationalize the OneHealth approach. The World Bank will support the establishment and/or strengthening of OneHealth platforms to facilitate cross-sectoral coop-eration and better advocacy across countries. At the level of the gov-ernment, policy recommendations for expanding overall government spending on health and other related sectors will include advocating for a specific line item financing allocation for disease surveillance, preparedness, and response, as well as contributions to ECOWAS to sustain regional networking arrangements for the long term. At the level of the development partners, the World Bank will explore via-ble options for diversifying the donor base, including the mobilization and the efficient and effective coordination of external resources for disease surveillance, epidemic preparedness, and rapid response in West Africa.

The Way Forward

The investment plans of Guinea, Liberia, and Sierra Leone offer a good start for moving toward a stronger health system, but this is only a start. More can and needs to be done. The countries' plans cover the essentials of a health strengthening effort, but it will be vital to ensure their imple-mentation through a plan that includes adequate, sustained resources.

The fiscal space analysis finds that, although governments must lever-age domestic resources to finance their health systems investment plans, sustained international support is going to be necessary to ensure that the plans are actually implemented. The main sources of increased fiscal space though domestic resources will be improved efficiency in the allocation and use of health sector resources, as well as a movement away from a reliance on direct, out-of-pocket payments to pooling and prepay-ment mechanisms in order to promote universal health coverage.

For all three countries, the specific interventions required to imple-ment the HRH plans should be guided by rigorous health education and health labor market assessments. Evidence from well-designed and repeated health training institution assessments is critical to identify existing capacity constraints and from health labor market assessments to identify the factors that motivate health workers to seek employment or perform better in a particular sector, type of health facility, or geographic location. Such assessments and evidence are absolutely essential to the design of targeted and effective policies that address prevailing problems. The mention of the importance of such studies in the investment plans of all three countries, in particular health labor market assessments, is a step in the right direction on this issue and needs to be supported by the World Bank immediately. This can be followed by collaborative efforts between the World Bank's Health and Education Department to consider relevant, strategically practical investments.

Reaching the targets identified in the investment plans will not substantially improve health worker densities, which is one vital area that must be addressed. A paradigm shift in *who* to train and *how* to train health workers is needed in all three countries. The focus in terms of HRH density needs to be primarily on innovative training policies, in particular rural pipeline policies, to scale up the rural health workforce. Moreover, any training efforts toward a fit-for-purpose health workforce should be combined with a continued focus on ensuring and improving capacities related to health worker performance.

Improved collaboration among countries in the form of a regional disease surveillance network is a critical step that will require strengthening cross-sectoral capacity as well as regional cooperation to earlier detect, better prepare, and rapidly respond to infectious diseases threats at the animal-human-ecosystem interface. This is an economically sound investment and a practical way to leverage resources to greater effect. Governments need to establish sustainable funding mechanisms for such a regional network.

Taken together, the issues addressed in this book provide compelling evidence that Guinea, Liberia, and Sierra Leone, working closely with the international community, have a historic opportunity to act in a manner that will go some distance toward mitigating the risks of global and regional epidemics. At the same time, acting on the recommendations put forward in this study should strengthen the health systems and ensure a reasonable level and quality of health care services in these countries, while also providing a roadmap for other developing countries that face similar situations.

The World Bank can be a key ally in this process by continuing to assist and work with Guinea, Liberia, and Sierra Leone in strengthening their health systems. Specifically, given the comparative advantage that it enjoys in the three areas addressed in this study, the World Bank can leverage its lending, knowledge, and convening power to provide, among other things, focused support to the three countries in the areas of health financing / fiscal space analysis, human resources for health, and disease surveillance and response.

Note

1. INAPs are country-owned action plans developed by countries affected and threatened by Avian and Human Influenza.

Reference

WHO (World Health Organization). 2016. *International Health Regulations (2005), 3rd ed*. Geneva: WHO.

National Investment Plans and Costing

This appendix presents the executive summaries of each country's investment plan. They are not entirely comparable, but they do provide an overview of their different approaches to investment costing and addressing fiscal space constraints.

Guinea Executive Summary

Sociopolitical and Economic Context

Despite the rich agricultural and mining potential of Guinea, its poverty has worsened since 1995 instead of improving. Indeed, Guinea is considered one of the poorest countries in West Africa. According to the poverty survey (*Enquête légère d'évaluation de la pauvreté*; ELEP) of 2012, just over 55 percent of the population live below the poverty line. This situation makes a good part of the population vulnerable and exposes it to catastrophic health expenditures (impoverishment), especially in a context where protection against the risk of disease is extremely low (less than 5 percent).

In 2014, per capita income (measured as gross domestic product) was about US$533, representing almost half the regional average. This level of income, coupled with negative per capita growth rates in 2014 and probably in 2015 (according to IMF data, 2015), does not reduce either the vulnerability or unemployment, or the bloated size, of the informal sector.

High population growth of Guinea highlights the challenges faced by the government to provide essential public services, including health. According to the General Population and Housing census of 2014,

Guinea has a population of 10.6 million inhabitants, with a density of about 41.4 inhabitants per square kilometer. Based on the rate of natural increase (2.38 percent), the Guinean population would be 13.5 million in 2024 (last year of the PNDS). The fertility rate, which is 5.1 children per woman, is higher than that of Sub-Saharan Africa (4.9 children per woman).

The country is urbanizing at a steady rate; the percentage of the urban population increased from 10 percent in 1960 to 30 percent in 2014. However, Conakry is the only city offering better access to services; the rest of the economy depends largely on the informal sector, with the majority of the population living in rural areas on subsistence agriculture. The agricultural sector is characterized by low productivity because it provides almost 80 percent of employment, but less than 20 percent of GDP.

In addition to the low level of education (34.5 percent), the economic vulnerability of households and the persistence of sociocultural taboos and some traditional standards have led to a reluctance to changes in behavior that would be conducive to good health.

After political instability marked by military hegemony, Guinea has engaged in a political and democratic process with a civilian government from 2010 (reinforced by the elections of October 2015). The period following this significant change has been characterized by a significant improvement in the macroeconomic situation and infrastructure. The country experienced significant growth between 2010 and 2012. However, in 2013, this growth slowed due to the cessation of investments in the mining sector and political unrest during the parliamentary elections. It was expected that growth would resume in 2014 and 2015. However, the Ebola epidemic, declared in March 2014, had a very negative impact, among others, on economic growth and sociosanitary situation.

In order to remedy this situation and strengthen the health system, the Government of the Republic of Guinea, with the support of its technical and financial partners, has initiated the development and implementation of a health system recovery plan for the years 2015–17, which is the first three-year plan to implement the National Health Development Plan (PNDS) from 2015 to 2024. A cost assessment process, PNDS financing and financial gaps, was also undertaken with the assistance of several technical and financial partners.

The total cost of the PNDS (2015–2024) is estimated at GNF 56,337 billion, about US$7,727,974,793. The cost per capita is estimated at US$57 in 2015 and will amount to US$74 in 2024. In the medium term, up to 2018, the average annual per capita cost will be just under US$60.

The difference between the available resources and estimated costs of the PNDS has permitted the identification of a total funding gap amounting to US$3.5 billion. This gap must be filled by a greater mobilization of domestic resources of the state and development partners. The low level of the gap in 2015 is explained by the existence of accurate data from partners for that year and also the commitments made by these same actors in the fight against the Ebola disease.

This costing exercise was to be accompanied by an analysis of fiscal space in order to better understand the opportunities and constraints associated with the mobilization of resources for the health sector. This exercise was conducted in the three affected countries hit by the Ebola virus (Guinea, Liberia, and Sierra Leone).

Definition and Methodology of the Analysis of Fiscal Space

The tax and fiscal space can be defined as the ability of a government to provide additional budgetary resources for a program or a sector without affecting the sustainability of the country's financial situation (Heller 2006).

The analysis of fiscal space tries to examine the possibility and the mechanism for a government to increase its spending in the short and medium terms in a manner consistent with the macroeconomic situation of the country (Tandon and Cashin 2010).

The fiscal space for the health sector could potentially be increased mainly through five sources (Heller 2006; Tandon and Cashin 2010):

a. Conducive macroeconomic conditions

b. Changing the order of priorities in the budget in favor of the sector

c. Increase of specific resources or dedicated to the sector

d. Additional resources mobilization as grants and / or loans

e. Efficiency gains

An Unfavorable Macroeconomic Situation

The economic situation in Guinea is unfavorable. The prospects for the medium and long terms are good enough but remain linked to many social and political internal factors (Ebola, postpresidential elections, and so on). Also to be noted are the importance of external threats to the Guinean economy such as lower commodity prices, the appreciation of the U.S. dollar, and rising interest rates.

This macroeconomic situation is not favorable to the enlargement of the fiscal space for health, especially in terms of allocation per capita in constant currency.

Expanding the Potential Fiscal Space through Earmarked Taxation and the Mobilization of External Funds

With the advent of Ebola—that has had a very negative impact on both the health of the population and the economy, in general, and public finances, in particular—the government put in place in 2015 two taxes on telephony: the Tax on Telephone Communications (TCT) and the Access Tax to the Telephone Network (TARTEL). TCT is a tax on consumption; it relates to telephone calls for which each second used is taxed up to GNF 1. During the month of August 2015, the amount of the TCT collected exceeded GNF 33 billion (DNI/DCS, September 2015). As for TARTEL, it taxes operators. These phone companies (four in number at present) pay 3 percent of their revenues in the framework of this new tax, which brought in to the state more than GNF 9 billion in August 2015 (DNI/DCS, September 2015).

This means that during a year, these two taxes could potentially bring to the state an amount more than GNF 510 billion (almost US$67 million). This amount is slightly higher than the budget allocated to health in fiscal year 2015 (GNF 492 billion).

With the aim of expanding the fiscal space, it would be appropriate to allocate all the mobilized annual amount from the new taxation on telephony to the health sector starting in fiscal year 2016.

In addition, the adoption of a universal health coverage policy to promote protection of the population against disease risks would be positive not only for improving the accessibility of the population to health care, but also to increase the fiscal space for health. One strategy would be to develop health insurance that would be a good way to channel mandatory contributions (contributions) to the health sector. This obviously implies substantially improving the level of the public health care providers.

The enlargement of the fiscal space is also possible through external funds. The health sector could benefit from a contribution of TFP up to US$35 per capita per year (against US$30 currently). However, this must be accompanied by a real external resource mobilization strategy and an improvement in the absorption capacity of the administration (health and other sectors) and its governance.

FIGURE A.1
Enlargement of Fiscal Space in Guinea, Possible Leeway

a. Options for Expanding the Health
Fiscal Space

Sources for the expansion of the fiscal space of the health sector in Guinea	Room to maneuver
Conducive macroeconomic conditions	Virtually zero
Changing the order of the budgetary priorities	Very high
Increase specific resources	High
Mobilize other resources : grants and loans	Pretty high
Efficiency gains	Very high

b. Magnitude of Expanding the Health
Fiscal Space, Different Sources

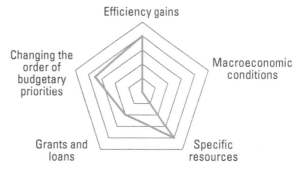

A Favorable Reprioritization in the Health Sector

Guinea could further expand the fiscal space of the health sector through a reprioritization within the state budget: the health sector could benefit from a greater share in the state budget of between 10 percent and 15 percent, against 3 percent today. This measure would be effective if the government implemented urgent measures to better implement the budget appropriations of the Ministry of Health.

Improving the Health Sector's Efficiency

Finally, the margin for the enlargement of the fiscal space of the health sector could come from improving the efficiency of the health sector. Compared to neighboring countries, the efficiency of the health sector in Guinea is below the subregional average. Guinea is not and will not even come near to achieving the health Millennium Development Goals (MDGs). This wide gap between goals and reality is mainly due to inefficiencies in the sector. This shift induced nearly 18,500 preventable deaths of mothers and children (respectively 1,500 and 17,000 in 2012), representing an economic loss equivalent to 4.8 percent of GDP (US$273 million).

Despite these efforts, a financial gap is observed between the financial resources of the state and its international partners on the one hand, and the costs for the PNDS for 2016–18, on the other hand. To fill it, the government and the donors should increase their contributions above 18.5 percent.

Quantitative Synthesis of the Analysis of Guinea's Fiscal Space in the Medium Term, 2016–18

Counting only the purely budgetary mobilization (improving efficiency is excluded) in the medium term, according to the proposals outlined above, the fiscal space for health in Guinea will have a significant impact on health financing (see table C.1), especially its public component. In effect:

- Public expenditures for health (DPS) will increase from US$5.7 per capita in 2015 to US$19.5 per capita in 2018.

- The ratio of these expenditures to GDP will be 2.8 percent in 2018, against 0.9 percent in 2015.

- The expense of technical and financial partners will increase from US$30.3 in 2015 to US$35 in 2018.

- The ratio of public spending to health spending in relation to TFP, which was 0.2 in 2015, will be 0.6 in 2018.

- Along with taxation on telephony and compulsory levies, the state must mobilize, in addition, US$3 per capita in 2017 and US$7 per capita in 2018 through a reprioritization policy.

TABLE A.1
Guinea: Evolution of Fiscal Space for Health in the Medium Term, 2015–18

Aspect of fiscal space	2015	2016	2017	2018
Public health expenditures per capita, US$	5.70	11.70	15.60	19.50
Public health expenditures per capita, GNF	43.492	89.269	118.727	148.409
Spending by technical and financial partners (TFP) per capita, US$	30,3	35,0	35,0	35,0
Public health expenditures / GDP	0,9%	1,9%	2,3%	2,8%
Public health expenditures / technical and financial partners (TFP) spending	0,2	0,3	0,4	0,6
Contribution of taxes on telephony and taxes per capita, US$		6	6,9	6,9
Contribution of reprioritization per capita, US$			3	6,9
A. Public health expenditures and technical and financial partners (TFP) spending per capita, US$	36	46.70	50.60	54.50
B. Cost of National Health Development plan per capita, US$	57	64,6	59	56,3
Gap: (A) – (B), US$	–21	–17.90	–8.40	–1.80

• Despite these efforts, a financial gap is observed between the financial resources of the state and its international partners on the one hand, and the costs for the PNDS for 2016–18. To fill this gap, the government and the donors should increase their contributions to above 18.5 percent.

Main Recommendations for the Enlargement of the Fiscal Space

Beyond the financial aspects of fiscal space, the report suggests the following recommendations:

• Engage in a universal health coverage process. The two biggest challenges at this level are: (i) the implementation of a plan to cover the poorest and most vulnerable in the Guinean population through public funds and (ii) the introduction of collective and strategic thinking about the possibilities to cover the informal sector.

• To achieve this, the government should take the following actions:

  ○ Undertake a study on the exact situation of health financing.

  ○ Define a health financing strategy and universal coverage policy.

  ○ Develop a law relating to universal health coverage.

  ○ Start the progressive implementation of universal health coverage policy.

  ○ Prepare the necessary implementing legislation and put in place the institutions and tools for the first steps toward universal health coverage.

• The state must make greater efforts to improve both its budgetary implementation capacity and the overall governance of the health system. Indeed, improving governance will give greater credibility to the health sector and other sectors that support it (including budget, finance, internal affairs, equipment, and the civil service). This represents the best advocacy for resource mobilization. In addition, the administration generally (because health does not depend only on the Ministry of Health) must also improve its capacity to absorb the available financial resources.

• Guinea should also significantly improve the efficiency of its health sector. This could be done through relevant measures, summarized as follows:

  ○ Reinvigorate and generalize a community approach (outreach).

  ○ Implement a new human resources policy targeting a wage increase; better basic and on the job training; better distribution in Guinea;

TABLE A.2
General Synthesis of the Analysis of Fiscal Space in Guinea

Elements of the fiscal space	Main points and observations	Recommendations	Scope
Macroeconomic context	The economic climate is unfavorable. The prospects for medium and long term are good enough but remain linked to many social and political internal factors (such as Ebola and post-presidential elections). Also noteworthy are external threats to the Guinean economy such as lower commodity prices, the appreciation of the U.S. dollar, and rising interest rates.	This macroeconomic situation is not favorable to the enlargement of the fiscal space for health, especially in terms of allocation per capita in constant currency.	No medium-term margin
Taxes dedicated to health	• Enlargement of the potential fiscal space through telephony related taxes: TCT and TARTEL • The establishment of CSU to promote protection of the population against the disease risk.	• Allocate the full annual amount of these taxes to health • Channel mandatory contributions to the health sector (with upgrade)	• GNF 510 billion or US$67 million annually from 2016 • Mobilized amount: GNF 156 billion from 2017. A good part could go to the public sector
External funds	Huge mobilization of technical and financial partners due to Ebola	The technical and financial partners must keep up their efforts, even in the post-Ebola period	It is possible and recommended that US$5 per capita be added, from 2016
Re-priorization	Despite the Ebola problem, the government allocates only 3% of its budget to health	Allocate between 10% and 15% instead of 3%	Gradually increase this allowance by 2 percentage points each year for 5 years
Improvement of the efficiency	• Compared to neighboring countries, the health sector is less efficient Guinea. • Guinea does not and will not even come near to achieve the health MDGs. This wide gap between goals and reality is mainly due to inefficiencies in the sector. • The shift induced nearly 18,500 preventable deaths of mothers and children (respectively, 1,500 and 17,000 in 2012), representing an economic loss equivalent to 4.8% of GDP (US$273 million).	Improve the efficiency of the health system: • Reinvigorate and generalize community approach (outreach) • A new human resources policy • A new policy for drugs' pricing, quality control, and regulation • Better management of resources • Gradually move toward universal health coverage. • Improved corporate governance • Implementation of a performance-based financing policy	This improvement would be much more efficient for the same budget and avoid the consequences in terms of avoidable casualties

an introduction of performance-based funding; regionalization of budget items.

o The Guinean health administration should be reviewed to ensure that each institution performs the functions for which it is created and does not abandon them to do the work of another institution. For example, the Medicines Directorate of the Ministry of Health must take care of pharmaceutical regulation and policy instead of playing the purchasing role at the central level, which should be played by the Central Pharmacy of Guinea (PCG).

o If it is indeed necessary for the Government of Guinea to significantly increase the extent of budget implementation dedicated to health, it must also improve the allocation of resources to high-impact and cost-effective interventions.

o Promotion of community health services adapted to the needs of the population. In this context, the decentralization policy (including fiscal decentralization) appears as a relevant policy for improving health sector performance.

o Once the sector improves (2016/17), it will become essential to think of developing and implementing a performance-based funding strategy (FBP) (starting with a pilot), where the efforts, resources, and attention are focused on results rather than inputs that are only a means and not a goal in themselves.

Liberia Executive Summary

1. In the last decade, Liberia had shown remarkable progress in rebuilding the health system from the devastation of the 14-year civil war. Strong results and progress toward meeting the Millennium Development Goals (MDGs) have been reported. For example, the proportion of deliveries attended by skilled health workers increased by about 60 percent, from 46 percent in 2007 to 73 percent in 2013; and immunization coverage more than doubled from 2007 to 2013, with the proportion of children having had a measles vaccination rising from 46 percent in 2007 to 73 percent in 2013; and measures of infant and childhood mortality also dropped significantly over the same period. These results were made possible through strong commitments by the Government of Liberia (GoL) and its development partners (DPs) to implement various sector development plans and programs. Furthermore, Liberia had already initiated steps toward achieving universal health coverage (UHC) in a proposal for the creation and

financing of the Liberia Health Equity Fund (LHEF). Design options and a roadmap for the LHEF have been drafted—proposing options intended to facilitate the financing and management of early phases of the initiative. The proposed design was costed, and possible sources of financing were also identified.

2. At the outbreak of the Ebola virus disease (EVD), in March 2014, Liberia had initiated an ambitious ten-year sector development plan that aimed to further strengthen the health system and consolidate the health gains from the previous five-year plan. Before EVD was contained, in May 2015, it had caused thousands of deaths, and had set back a decade of progress of building up the health system.

3. Despite evident progress, the health system continues to face significant challenges and remains poorly equipped to effectively respond to epidemics with adequate safety and infection control measures as well as safe and effective service provision. Among the system's prominent problems were insufficient numbers of, and poorly motivated, health workers; insufficient and nonfunctioning equipment; weak supply chains, poor logistical support; and poor quality of care.

4. Total health expenditures (THE) have seen a marked increase over the last decade, increasing from US$100 million in 2007/08 to over US$365 million in 2013/14, as reported in a series of National Health Accounts (NHA). Despite the fact that the GoL budget allocation has been increasing over the years (reaching 12 percent of the total GoL budget in FY2014/15), it remains a small proportion of the THE. External donors and households—through out-of-pocket payment—are the two main sources of financing, each accounting for about 40 percent of THE. Although the exact amount is difficult to establish, it is well known that a substantial portion of the external financing is provided "off-budget" through NGOs directly to counties and communities. A recent donor mapping exercise by MoH has estimated that close to three-fourths of donor funding is channeled through "off-budget" mechanisms.

5. The health sector encounters two critical challenges related to budget execution and allocation, among others:

   • Health budget executions have been consistently lower than the amount allotted (appropriated by parliament). Multiple causes are identified for the inability of MoH to spend allotted amounts; many of them pertain to broader PFM challenges across the GoL. Weak execution within the health sector is problematic in and of itself, as unspent resources do not go to service provision and/or are spent hastily at the end of the fiscal year.

- The absence of transparent and objective resource allocation criteria has resulted in an inequitable distribution of the health budget across counties. To address this issue, a resource allocation formula was developed by MoH a couple of years ago. However, due to the lack of information on "off-budget" donor funding, MoH has encountered practical challenges in applying the formula. Among other issues, the absence of objective resource allocation criteria makes it difficult to attempt any kind of efficiency analyses. It will be critical that MoH to continue its efforts: first, to capture the off-budget donor funding through a comprehensive donor mapping exercise; and second, to progressively align the off-budget funding through improved sector coordination and formalizing the aid effectiveness principles through the IHP+.

6. As the EVD crisis started to recede, Liberia's Ministry of Health, working in collaboration with DPs, developed an "Investment Plan for Building a Resilient Health System, 2015–21, a seven-year plan. The investment plan is designed to address three high-priority thematic areas: (i) build a fit-for-purpose productive and motivated health workforce that equitably and optimally delivers quality services; (ii) reengineer the health infrastructure to conform to the population's needs for health services; and (iii) strengthen epidemic preparedness surveillance and response, including the expansion of the established surveillance and early warning and response system to ensure that it is comprehensive enough to detect and respond to future health threats to the public. It further identifies nine priority investment areas.

7. The investment plan is costed using an ingredient costing approach. The costing and financing gap analysis presents three scenarios. These scenarios call for a substantially higher level of investment compared to what Liberia has been investing in health thus far. The best case scenario asks for a total cost of US$1.73 billion over the seven years, with a financing gap estimated at US$757 million—it considers all ideal interventions proposed to build a resilient health system. The moderate case scenario projects a total cost of US$1.61 billion and a financing gap estimated at US$641 million—it includes interventions that should be implemented to build a more resilient health system. The baseline case scenario estimates a total cost of US$1.06 billion and a financing gap of US$90 million—it captures interventions that are critical to build a resilient health system.

8. Given the large amount of resources that will be needed to realize the goals of the investment plan, it has become necessary to analyze all

sources from which funds could be mobilized. This book is written with the objective of exploring the degree to which additional fiscal space for health can be created to contribute to the resources needed. Building on prior work by MoH, and complemented with a global database, the analysis looks into five possible sources of fiscal space for health: (i) rates of economic growth and increases in government revenue to assess the fiscal context for increased allocations for health; (ii) the feasibility of increasing health budgets by reprioritizing health, relative to other sectors, in the national budget; (iii) the feasibility of raising additional domestic revenue for health through increased taxation, including an earmarked tax; (iv) potential gains that might be found through improved allocations and technical efficiency in the health sector; and (v) the potential for improved mobilization of external resources.

9. This book analyzes the five potential sources for increased fiscal space for health in Liberia. Projected fiscal space and the financing gap for the implementation of the investment plan are summarized in the table below. Two scenarios are considered in generating the projected figures. These are the key points for each funding source:

- *Increased government budget*—faster economic growth and reprioritization of health within the government budget. Reaching the "Abuja Target" of devoting 15 percent of total government allocations to health will necessarily require concomitant reductions in allocations to other sectors. While achieving this high target (current allocations have only approached 12 percent) is basically a political decision, support for it can be strengthened by more efficient use of existing allocations to health and of current external assistance amounts. Conclusive evidence of significant economic returns to added investments in the health sector needs to be developed and used in advocacy for this fiscal space expansion through reprioritization.

- *An increase in health-sector-specific resources*—through earmarked or other taxation that could be allocated to the health budget, such as "sin" taxes on alcoholic beverages and tobacco products, surcharges on automobile registration fees or on automobile insurance, and levies on airline tickets or on international departures, a portion of value-added tax (VAT) transferred to health (2 to 3 percent). While "sin" taxes are conducive to healthful behavior, they are unlikely to generate much revenue for health. The same may also be true of taxes on vehicle registration. Moreover, a VAT has not yet been introduced in Liberia. When implemented, it is likely to be assessed on a

· smaller basket of goods and services, since it would be regressive, and thus likely to be paid by those who can least afford to pay the tax. The VAT and contributions through payroll taxes should be further explored as part of a proper actuarial analysis for the LHEF.

• *Increases in health-sector-specific grants and foreign aid:* The government has little control over the level and trends of financial and/or project assistance from external sources—especially in a situation where the "off-budget" amounts are substantially in excess of the "on-budget" amounts. In such an environment, the focus of government advocacy should be, at least, to maintain current levels, and, whenever possible, to invest efforts and resources in advocating how increased external aid can and will be efficiently used by MoH and by the counties to improve population health status.

• *An increase in the efficiency of existing government outlays* in all sectors: National Health Accounts estimates show that there are substantial resources devoted to the health sector—dominated largely by external assistance, both "off-budget" and "on-budget" categories. In this context, there are ample opportunities to stretch existing funding to finance a larger amount of services. Finding such opportunities is not easy, and capturing the savings for expanding service delivery is even more difficult. A fundamental prerequisite for expanding fiscal space through greater efficiency (focusing on both technical and allocative efficiency) is to inject greater equity in the process of allocating funds among the counties.

Priority Recommended Activities

1. *Boost coordinated, increased funding from DPs:* Both the Aid Management Unit (in MoFDP) and the External Aid Coordination Unit (in MoH) should be given more resources and more authority to perform their functions—to require donors and NGOs to register as development partners and to design their programs to be explicitly supportive of MoH's policies and programs. Specifically, MoH should require partners to share budgets and work plans each year as prerequisite for being reregistered as an NGO and receive approval to work in Liberia's health sector. Currently, MoFDP's Aid Management Unit (AMU), which relies on voluntary reporting, and the National Health Accounts estimates, which rely on surveys of DP spending, are the only entities estimating the magnitude of "off-budget" activities. DPs should be encouraged to test alternative program approaches to increase efficiency in health services delivery through performance-based

TABLE A.3
Liberia: Projected Total Fiscal Space for the Health and Financing Gap
U.S. dollars, millions

Aspect of scenario	2015/16	2016/17	2017/18	2018/19	2019/20	2020/21	2021/22
Scenario 1							
Total fiscal space for health	200.56	161.13	148.93	148.48	159.52	167.29	160.13
Government budget for health	74.11	82.15	81.87	83.42	94.45	102.19	115.88
Sin taxes on alcohol and tobacco	0.72	0.79	0.86	0.94	1.02	1.12	1.22
Motor vehicle taxes and fees	0.86	0.91	0.96	1.02	1.08	1.15	1.22
External resources	124.87	77.28	65.24	63.10	62.96	62.83	41.81
Cost of investment plan							
Best case scenario	217.73	224.30	218.44	219.58	247.30	269.26	280.62
Moderate case scenario	202.12	208.93	203.67	205.72	227.98	251.12	257.89
Base case scenario	137.42	129.33	131.05	137.89	147.50	157.26	165.94
Financing gap							
Best case scenario	17.17	63.17	69.51	71.10	87.78	101.98	120.49
Moderate case scenario	1.56	47.80	54.74	57.25	68.46	83.83	97.76
Base case scenario	(63.14)	(31.79)	(17.88)	(10.59)	(12.02)	(10.03)	5.81
Scenario 2							
Total fiscal space for health	202.28	202.40	199.16	198.19	202.28	202.26	209.72
Government budget for health	74.11	89.00	95.51	104.27	118.06	127.74	144.85
Sin taxes on alcohol and tobacco	1.45	1.58	1.72	1.88	2.05	2.23	2.43
Motor vehicle taxes and fees	1.72	1.82	1.93	2.05	2.17	2.30	2.44
External resources	125.00	110.00	100.00	90.00	80.00	70.00	60.00
Cost of investment plan							
Best case scenario	217.73	224.30	218.44	219.58	247.30	269.26	280.62
Moderate case scenario	202.12	208.93	203.67	205.72	227.98	251.12	257.89
Base case scenario	137.42	129.33	131.05	137.89	147.50	157.26	165.94
Financing gap							
Best case scenario	15.45	21.90	19.27	1.39	45.02	67.00	70.90
Moderate case scenario	(0.15)	6.53	4.51	7.53	25.70	48.85	48.17
Base case scenario	(64.85)	(73.06)	(68.12)	(60.31)	(54.77)	(45.00)	(43.78)

financing methods, and to exchange information on results and best practices in PBF.

2. *Strengthen MoH leadership through the Health Sector Coordination Committee (HSCC)*: Revive and strengthen the health sector coordination, accountability, and alignment effort. For a start, the HSCC can act as a coordinating mechanism to rally all DPs around the investment plan and aim to strengthen the efficiency of "off-budget" funds. A strengthened HSCC should be empowered to make decisions on (i) the reallocation/ redirection of funds to priority areas, (ii) prioritization of the investment plan, (iii) directing partner resources to MoH priority areas, and (iv) reducing duplicative activities.

3. *Introduce transparent and objective resource allocation criteria for the health sector.* This will require MoH to carry out a comprehensive resource mapping exercise to fully capture donor funding, particularly the portion channeled through "off-budget" channels.

4. *Engage MoFDP to address PFM issues.* It has been documented that MoH receives (i.e., spends) about three-fourths of total budgeted amounts in any given fiscal year. While the funds may ultimately be made available and spent, if carried over to subsequent fiscal years, the associated loss of staff time and promptness of receipts hampers the efficient delivery of services.

Sierra Leone Executive Summary

This section reviews the performance of the Sierra Leone health sector and identifies how the country can increase its fiscal space to address its health and social challenges, poverty, and inequality. The study identifies that the Government of Sierra Leone's current health budget is below 10 percent of the total government budget, which is less when compared to the Abuja target of 15 percent of total government budget. In per capita terms, the government of Sierra Leone's average health expenditures between 2010 and 2013 were US$6.10, which was well below the US$34 recommended by WHO's Commission on Macroeconomics. The study also identifies that the bulk of health financing over the years has come from out-of-pocket expenses, which has the tendency to prevent access, and in others to impose severe financial stress on people using services. This method of financing the health sector also encourages inefficiency and inequity in the way available resources are used, by exacerbating overservicing for people who can pay, accompanied by underservicing for people who cannot. Donor funding has also remained critical in health sector financing.

As the country is vigorously engaged in driving the Ebola epidemic to an end, a comprehensive response focused on contract tracing, disease surveillance, and community engagement has been established by the government with support from key stakeholders. The GoSL, with support from development partners, has developed a Health Strengthening Strategy (HSS) plan with an estimated cost of US$487.84 million to fully finance activities in the plan for 2016, 2017, and 2018. With regard to funding, so far donors have sent in information on their planned expenditures to the tune of US$298 million for 2016 and 2017. About US$63 million of that is, however, pegged to emergency food aid. Thus, the planned expenditures for funding the five pillars of the HSS plan amount to US$231million for the two years. This gives a resource gap of US$256.84 million for the three years. This financing gap has created demands for additional fiscal space for the health sector. The study estimates that inclusive of external funding, there is a potential to generate revenue of US$180.30 million, US$223.67 million, and US$204.80 million in 2016, 2017, and 2018, respectively, to support the health HSS plan for the three years in Sierra Leone.

The study notes that the macroeconomic projections (in the short and medium terms), which determine how much a country can spend in the future, are not very promising; and coupled with the declining priority for health in the government budget, the potential for additional fiscal space for health is greatly impaired. Other potential sources of additional resources for fiscal space identified in this study—including increased domestic revenue mobilization, earmarking tax revenue from the sale of tobacco, and the introduction of a social health insurance scheme—all have got their own challenges and would require strong state institutions and political will.

Therefore, external assistance in the health sector remains very critical in the short and medium terms (post-Ebola) for ensuring a resilient health system in Sierra Leone. The study also admonishes that it would be unethical to argue for increased government funding of the health sector if the resources are not used either efficiently or equitably. The study identifies the sources of inefficiencies, in particular leakages out of the health system due to the fragmented payment system, charging of illegal fees, and procurement management of medicines and supplies. The study concludes that the main priority for increasing fiscal space in Sierra Leone is to address the underlying inefficiencies which constrain current fiscal space, and intervention by development partners to reverse the poor health service delivery outcomes that have been exacerbated by the EVD outbreak.

References

Heller, Peter S. 2005. "Understanding Fiscal Space." IMF Policy Discussion Paper, PDP/05/4, International Monetary Fund, Washington, DC.

Tandon, Ajay, and Cheryl Cashin. 2010. "Assessing Public Expenditure on Health from a Fiscal Space Perspective." Health, Nutrition, and Population Discussion Paper, World Bank, Washington, DC.

Components of Investment Plans and Fiscal Space Projections for the Health Workforce

TABLE B.1.1

Proposed Interventions in Country Investment Plans for Workforce Scaling Up and Distribution

Guinea (2015–17)	Priorities/focus	Proposed interventions
	By 2017, to increase density, motivation, and equitable distribution of human resources for health	• Recruitment of health workforce—about 2,000 every year • Ensure salaries of existing staff, including new recruits, and a 40% rise in Ministry of Health staff salaries • Retain and redeploy staff currently hired to fight Ebola (about 2,000) • Update HRH plan based on PNDS • Set up human resources information systems • Develop national harmonized standards for training (initial and continuous) and plan for continuing education • Study labor market and staff productivity • Establish effective system of incentives and allocation of staff to underserved areas • Establish system of recruitment and motivation • Cost implications: US$94.8 million (2015–17)

table continues next page

TABLE B.1.1

Proposed Interventions in Country Investment Plans for Workforce Scaling Up and Distribution *(continued)*

Liberia (2015–21)	Priorities/focus	Proposed interventions
	Needs-based recruitment and retention and address maldistribution	• Emergency health workforce hiring to restore essential services and core health system functions • Validate and clean the Government of Liberia's payroll and ensure equitable payment across professions/levels • Absorb 4,132 public sector health workers not on payroll • Implement housing allowance policy for 10% of the workforce in the most underserved areas • Reduce attrition by developing fair and equitable remuneration (hardship allowance), social protection, and retirement benefits • Establish mobile money platform for timely remuneration • Recruit health workers for additional facilities Focal health worker cadres for scaling up • Community health workers (CHW) • Health managers • Registered nurses (including nurse specialists) • Registered midwives • Physicians (including specialists)
	Innovative strategies to improve health worker performance and accountability	• Rapid action plan to be developed and implemented for in-service training, supportive supervision, and quality improvement • Regulatory campus to strengthen regulatory systems
	Strengthen training and education at preservice level and postgraduate education	• Hardship and merit-based scholarships for currently enrolled students to reduce dropout rates • Improve quality of existing preservice training programs to address the range of skills required (physicians, nurses, midwives, managers, community health workers), infrastructure upgrades, faculty recruitment, and curriculum review • Seed funding to establish new preservice education programs through public-private partnerships • Enhance West Africa's regional collaboration arrangements to strengthen training institutional capacity
	Standardize and scale up community health worker (CWH) programs to deliver basic health services in rural areas	• Pilot and evaluate production and implementation of CWH programs for communities more than 5 kilometers from health facilities (approximately 29% of total population) • Update existing community health policy and roadmap—begin recruiting, training, and supervising CWHs in selected counties

table continues next page

TABLE B.1.1

Proposed Interventions in Country Investment Plans for Workforce Scaling Up and Distribution
(continued)

	Ensure robust, long-term, needs-based health workforce planning, management, and development	• Reform of Ministry of Health HRH structure • Strengthen health worker information system, including validation of remaining 3,000/11,000 records in iHRIS • Complete health workforce census and analysis of health workforce needs • Develop strategy based on study to address health workforce motivation • Build cycles of regular evidence-based and needs-informed workforce planning • Cost implications: US$510.6 million (2015–21; best case scenario)
Sierra Leone (2015–20)	**Priorities/focus**	**Proposed interventions**
	Increase skilled workforce with an emphasis on underserved areas and community-based delivery	• Redeploy the 40–50% clinical MOHS staff and 30–40% skilled volunteers, and 15–20% unskilled volunteers who will be affected by the closure of Ebola facilities • In the short run, fast-track recruitment of Sierra Leone health workers abroad • Integrate and institutionalize the CHW cadre within MoHS • Review of HRH policy, update remuneration packages, and incentives, including further rollout of performance-based financing pilot. Include definitions of "hard to reach" and "remote" to determine appropriate incentives.
	Establish and deliver in-service health worker training package for Sierra Leone Basic Package of Essential Health Services (BPEHS)	• Establish 3 regional hubs as centers of excellence to train health workers and serve as referral hubs; these will develop quality-of-care guidelines, mentor local practitioners, and provide training and emergency high-level care. • Establish continuing education programs
	Establish a local postgraduate medical training program	• To ensure production of sufficient specialists • Cost implications: US$222.2 million (2015–20; aggressive scenario)

TABLE B.1.2
Budget Forecast, Workforce Cost, and Projections, 2014, 2020, and 2030

	Projection	Workforce cost (US$, millions)[a]	GDP (US$, millions)	GDP (%)	Government expenditures (US$, millions)	Government expenditures (%)	Health expenditures (US$, millions)[b]	Health expenditures (%)
Guinea	Current[b]	11.8	6,699	0.18%	1,775.24	0.66%	65.15	18%
	Total workforce with scaling up (2020)[a]	17.5	8,765	0.20%	2,427.91	0.72%	89.10	20%
	Plan doctors, nurses, and midwives; total cost, 2020[c]	10.4	8,765	0.12%	2,427.91	0.43%	89.10	12%
	2.5/1,000 population doctors, nurses, and midwives; total cost, 2020[c]	15.9	8,765	0.18%	2,427.91	0.65%	89.10	18%
	2.5/1,000 population doctors, nurses, and midwives; total cost, 2029 (at 2020 national data projections)[c]	74.3	8,765	0.85%	2,427.91	3.06%	89.10	83%
	On the basis of 5% growth rate, 2020–30	74.3	14,277	0.52%	3,954.79	1.88%	145.14	51%
Liberia	Current[b]	37	2,012	1.84%	645.85	5.73%	80.1	46%
	Total wage bill with scaling up (2020)[a]	48.8	3,011	1.62%	909.32	5.37%	112.76	43%
	Plan doctors, nurses, and midwives; total cost, 2020[c]	44.9	3,011	1.49%	909.32	4.94%	112.76	40%
	2.5/1,000 population nurses, and midwives; total cost, 2020[c]	27.2	3,011	0.90%	909.32	2.99%	112.76	24%

2.5/1,000 population doctors, nurses and midwives total cost 2029 (at 2020 national data projections)[c]	69	3,011	2.29%	909.32	7.59%	112.76	61%
On the basis of 5% growth rate, 2020–30	69	4,905	1.41%	1,481.19	4.66%	183.67	38%
Sierra Leone — Current[b]	31.2	4,746	0.66%	859.026	3.63%	60.99	51%
Total wage bill with scaling up, 2020[a]	90.3	5,034	1.79%	906.12	9.97%	64.33	140%
Plan doctors, nurses, and midwives; total cost, 2020[c]	116.9	5,034	2.32%	906.12	12.90%	64.33	182%
2.5/1000 population doctors, nurses, and midwives; total cost, 2020[c]	75.9	5,034	1.51%	906.12	8.38%	64.33	118%
2.5/1000 population doctors, nurses, and midwives; total cost 2029 (at 2020 national data projections)[c]	462.3	5,034	9.18%	906.12	51.02%	64.33	719%
On the basis of 5% growth rate, 2020–30	462.3	8,200	5.64%	1,475.97	31.32%	104.79	441%

Source: International Monetary Fund, World Economic Outlook Database, April 2016.

a. Costs for "scenario 2" are used for all workforce costs.

b. Current estimates are based on 2016 cost projections compared to 2014 levels of GDP, government expenditures and government expenditures on health using government expenditures on health as a percentage of total government expenditures; 3.67 percent for Guinea, 12.4 percent for Liberia, and 7.1 percent for Sierra Leone. 2020 estimates are calculated using target percentages discussed in government fiscal space publications.

c. Total cost estimates for doctors, nurses, and midwives represent those at progress toward target 2020 and 2029. For 2.5/1,000 population projection, the target date used is 2030.

Analysis of Health Workforce Targets Derived from the Costing of Those Targets

Introduction

Whereas the main report focuses on the HRH density targets outlined in the investment plans, this separate analysis assesses the targets extracted from the costing exercise. The implications of these targets are assessed in relation to projected population growth, graduate production, and cost.

The costing plans in each of the three countries stipulate the total number (and cost) of health workers to be trained over the next 6 to 10 years. While Guinea and Sierra Leone have projected scaling-up plans until 2024 and 2025, respectively, Liberia has projected scaling-up plans until 2021. The rationale behind the training of health workers varies depending on the country (with no rationale listed for Guinea). Furthermore, not all cadre targets were included in all countries and costed in the exercise (notably in Guinea and Sierra Leone). In discussions with relevant country counterparts, it was agreed to assume 100 percent scaling-up assumptions for those cadres for which targets had not been inserted in the costing exercise (this was considered an input error). An overview of the costing plans and terms of the planned scaling up in each of the three countries, as well as the rationale behind the training scaling-up plans and some of the assumptions on the scaling-up of some cadres, are provided in table B.2.1.

Scaling-Up Plans According to Costing Tools

All three countries are proposing to more than double their health workforce; this translates into ambitious annual increases in health

TABLE B.2.1
Costing Plan Target Details and Assumptions, by Country

Aspect of plan	Guinea	Liberia	Sierra Leone
Source	OneHealth Tool	Costing Health Investment Case & Plan_2015_v.45(27 Oct)	Basic Package of Essential Health Services (BPEHS)_HRH Staffing levels – 22 Mar 15
Terms of planned scaling up	Specific number of trainees to be trained each year up to 2024	Total number of trainees to be trained by 2021	Gap between BPEHS and current stock
Rationale behind scaling-up plan	Unknown	Number of health workers required for new and upgraded facilities and specialist training funded by the Health Workforce Program	HRH staffing norms for health facilities as of 2014
Cadres for which target not available and 100 percent scaling up is assumed (based on government consultations)	• Specialists • Logistics • Public health nurse • Administrative support • Other/assistant health professional	• Health care assistant • Health support • Administrative support • Logistics • Dentists (50 percent scaling up)	None

workers trained. Table B.2.2 provides a picture of the current stock of the health workforce (reflecting 2015 payroll data) and planned scaling-up targets.[1] The average annual percentage increase was then calculated. Accordingly, Guinea is planning a 10.3 percent annual increase of its overall health workforce, closely followed by Liberia (9.5 percent), and finally Sierra Leone (8 percent).

Although all three countries emphasize the scaling up of high-level cadres, countries vary in their emphasis on mid- and lower-level cadres. As shown in table B.2.2, according to the target numbers of health cadres to be produced, Liberia has emphasized the scaling up of high-level workers' (physicians) cadres and midwives. Guinea's greatest emphasis is mid-level workers (nurses and midwives), though high-level (physicians) are also a focus. Sierra Leone is focusing on scaling up high-level workers (general practitioners and specialists) as well as some low-level cadres (nurse and midwife associates, medical and laboratory technicians); and Liberia and Sierra Leone have emphasized cadres for scaling-up in which they already have a larger stock position (mid level in Liberia and low level in Sierra Leone). While the costing tool did set some targets for CHWs, the different definitions of CHWs (from volunteers to frontline civil servants) made comparison of numbers between the three countries not feasible).

TABLE B.2.2

2015 Stock of Health Workforce, by Cadre and Planned Scaling Up from Costing Tools

Percent annual growth

Cadre	Guinea		Liberia		Sierra Leone	
	2015	2024	2015	2021	2015	2025
Total	6,961	16,949 (10.3%)	11,233	19,465 (9.5%)	11,060	24,057 (8%)
High level (doctors)	1,111	2,810 (10.8%)	158	341 (13.7%)	234	705 (11.6%)
Mid level	1,735	7,424 (17.5%)	3,474	6,115 (9.9%)	768	1,726 (8.4%)
Low level	4,115	6,715 (5.6%)	7,601	13,009 (9.3 %)	9,253	21,626 (8.8%)
Nurses	1,168	4,976 (17.4%)	2,445	3,625 (6.8%)	450	1,090 (9.2%)
Midwives	372	2,269 (22.2%)	952	2,378 (16.4%)	208	508 (9.2%)

Note: The 2015 stock is reflected in the payroll for all countries. Health staff have been categorized as high (general practitioners and specialist doctors), mid (registered nurses, midwife professionals, and others), and low (medical assistants and others). Community health workers are not included in the low-level cadre categorization.

Implications of Scaling-Up Plans for Health Worker Density

The following assesses the picture of how proposed scaling-up plans in each of the three countries translate into health worker densities when taking into account population growth projections. Table B.2.3 provides an overview of how health worker densities were calculated.

Taking into account population growth projections shows that scaling-up plans are much more modest in outcome than the proposed increase in numbers suggests. Figure B.2.1(a) shows that scaling-up targets translate into overall improvements of densities of similar magnitude, with Sierra Leone achieving bigger increases in staff density than the other two. Also evident, however, is that overall increases in staff densities are limited. By the end of its plan, Guinea, which starts from an extremely low level, will not even reach the current density of Sierra Leone; and by the end of its plan, Sierra Leone will just reach the current density of Liberia. This means that health worker density levels will still remain low even if targets are reached as planned.

TABLE B.2.3
Calculation Methods of Health Worker Densities

Aspect of method	Guinea	Liberia	Sierra Leone
How "trainees per year" was calculated	Added the number of trainees to the current (2015) stock reflected by the payroll	Determined the gap between the 2021 target and current (2015) stock and spread this gap evenly between 2015 and 2021	Determined the gap between the BPEHS requirement and the current (2015) stock reflected by the payroll and spread the number evenly between 2015 and 2025
How "densities per year" was calculated	Scaling-up numbers by year were imposed with population growth projections	Scaling-up numbers by year were imposed with population growth projections	Scaling-up numbers by year were imposed with population growth projections

Note: BPESH = Basic Package of Essential Health Services.

FIGURE B.2.1
Workforce Scaling-Up Implications for Density, by Country

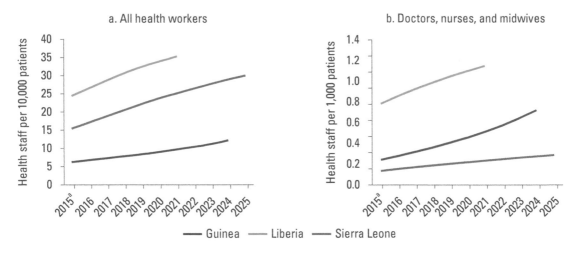

a. Current stock.

Comparing doctor, nurses, and midwife densities, it is evident that the proposed scaling-up targets will get the three Ebola-affected countries nowhere near commonly recommended density thresholds. Indeed, neither the old density threshold of 2.28 doctors, nurses, and midwives per 1,000 population, which is associated with service delivery coverage, nor the new density threshold of 4.45 doctors, nurses, and midwives, which is associated with achieving universal health coverage on HRH, will be anywhere met. Sierra Leone in particular will show limited progress on this front, as seen in figure B.2.1(b).

Implications of Scaling-Up Plans for Skill Mix Densities

This section examines, at a high level, the variation in the investment emphasis that scaling-up plans place on the scaling up of a crude classification of the different categories of health cadres (high, medium, and low). The type of cadre on which to focus has implications for both costs and for service delivery needs.

Among the three countries, Guinea plans the largest relative increase in its high-level cadres, despite already having the highest baseline. As seen in figure B.2.2, the largest relative increase of doctors (both general practitioners and specialists) is planned in Guinea, for an increase in staff density from 0.1 to 0.2 doctors per 1,000 population by 2024. This is despite the fact that, of all three countries, Guinea already has by far the largest number of high-level cadres. By the end of their proposed scaling-up efforts, neither Sierra Leone nor Liberia would reach the density levels for high-level cadres that Guinea already has today. It is important to note that Liberia's plan has a shorter time frame (to 2021), and its trajectory for higher-level cadres tracks that of Sierra Leone.

Guinea is planning the largest proportional increase of mid-level cadres, although densities of these workers will fall significantly short of those currently experienced by Liberia. Liberia has the largest numbers (and highest density) of mid-level workers and is planning a large increase. As seen in figure B.2.3 for mid-level cadres, Guinea

FIGURE B.2.2
Scaling Up of High-Level Cadres, by Country

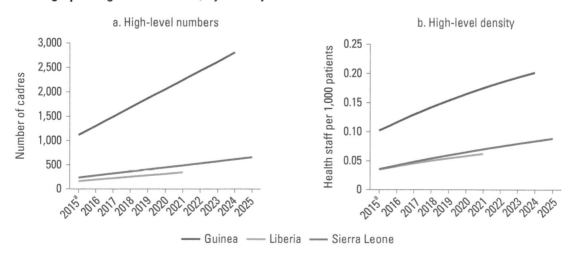

a. Current stock.

FIGURE B.2.3
Scaling Up of Mid-Level Cadres, by Country

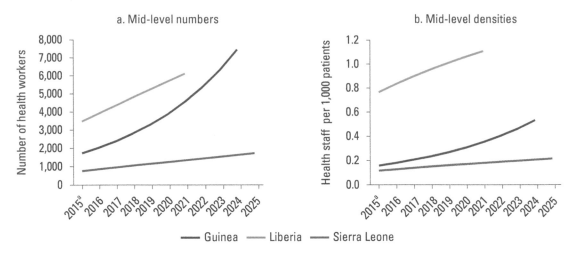

a. Current stock.

is planning to increase mid-level workers more than the other two countries, although its density per 1,000 workers falls short of achieving Liberia's density. Sierra Leone has the lowest availability and is planning a very small scaling up both in terms of headcount and density.

Sierra Leone is planning the largest increase in low-level cadres among the three countries and will meet Liberia's density distribution, whereas Guinea will fall far behind in this area. Figure B.2.4 shows that Guinea has planned a very small increase in this cadre, with density levels remaining low in 2024. Again, it is important to note the shorter time frame for Liberia; its trajectory for lower-level cadres falls somewhere between that of Guinea and Sierra Leone over the 2015–21 period.

Implications of Scaling-Up Plans for Actual Graduate Production and Cost

This section considers the implications of the proposed scaling-up plans for the actual number and cost of trainees required each year when taking into account different scenarios of attrition and employment rates. The costing plans list and cost the number of health workers to train (and their targets, which are analyzed above), but these numbers do not take into account possible levels of attrition and employment rates that are common in each country. Given the absence of actual comparable data on workforce attrition, training dropout rates, and employment rates,

FIGURE B.2.4
Scaling Up of Low-Level Cadres, Headcount, and Densities, by Country

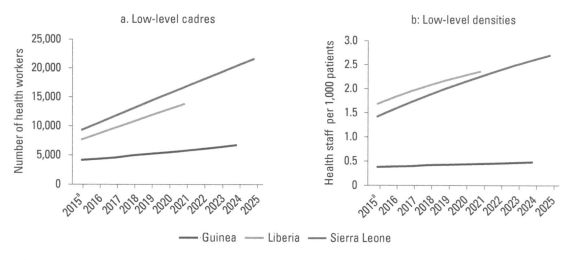

a. Low-level cadres

b: Low-level densities

— Guinea — Liberia — Sierra Leone

a. Current stock.

TABLE B.2.4
Three Scenarios of Attrition and Employment That Affect Scaling-Up Plans
Percent

Scenario	Workforce attrition	Drop out of training	Employment rate
Base scenario	0	0	100
Scenario 1	5	10	75
Scenario 2	10	20	50

three common theoretical scenarios were generated taking these variables into account (table B.2.4). The base scenario is the most optimistic yet unrealistic scenario, which reflects the training numbers in the scaling-up plans.

When different forms of attrition, dropout rates, and employment rates are taken into account, the number of annual graduates required to meet scaling-up targets for different cadres is significantly higher. It would have large implications for the number of enrollment places required for different health worker cadres. Figure B.2.5 shows the impact of the different scenarios for nurses in Guinea. The relative impact is proportionately identical for all cadres in all three countries under identical assumptions about workforce losses that result from the three causes (attrition, dropping out, and a fall in the employment rate).

FIGURE B.2.5

Number of Trainees Required to Meet Targets for Nurses in Guinea, by Scenario

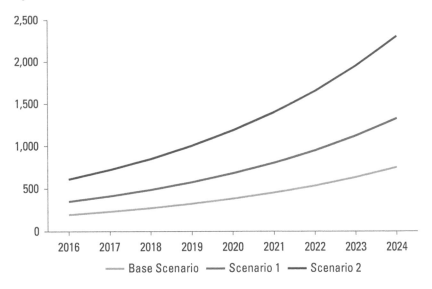

Once attrition, dropout rates, and employment rates are taken into account, costs are also significantly higher than estimated by the base scenario. Table B.2.5 provides a breakdown of costs by health workforce categorization (high, middle, and low cadres) for the base scenario and the scenarios that take into account the extra costs associated with training additional health workers to allow for attrition, dropout, and employment uptake rates and still meet the desired workforce target. For each country, costs were calculated until the year indicated in its scaling-up plan. Some assumptions used in the cost projections are:

• Total costs include salary and training costs

• The average salary reflected in the payroll is used

• Where the training cost is not known, the training cost for a staff group with similar earnings is used

Since additional costs relate entirely to those of training (each scenario achieves the same health workforce stock, so the costs of paying that stock do not vary by scenario), the rate of increase depends on the relative cost levels of training and pay. Such costs are much higher in Sierra Leone than they are in Guinea or Liberia (see below), so the impact of increasing attrition and dropout and reducing employment uptake are correspondingly greater. Scenarios 1 and 2 increase annual labor force costs by 12 and 16 percent, respectively, in Guinea or Liberia; in Sierra Leone this increase is 32 and 34 percent, respectively.

TABLE B.2.5

Annual Cost Implications of Scaling Up and Additional Training, by Country and Scenario

U.S. dollars, millions

Country (end year of scaling-up plan)	Scenario	High-level cadre	Mid-level cadre	Low-level cadre	Total
Guinea (2024)	Base scenario	3.9	10.2	6.5	20.6
	Scenario 1	4.6	11.7	6.8	23.1
	Scenario 2	5.5	14.2	7.3	27.0
Liberia (2021)	Base scenario	2.5	16.1	20.8	39.5
	Scenario 1	3.2	18.3	22.9	44.4
	Scenario 2	4.4	21.5	25.8	51.8
Sierra Leone (2024)	Base scenario	15.2	8.4	51.5	75.1
	Scenario 1	20.8	10.9	67.8	99.5
	Scenario 2	28.9	14.5	90.8	134.1

In summary, once market factor assumptions such as attrition, training dropout, and employment rates in the public sector are taken into consideration, training capacity required to produce the desired number of health staff, as well as the associated costs, increase. Relatively modest and uniform rates of attrition, dropout,[2] and employment across all cadres are used to demonstrate the effect of taking these factors into consideration. In reality, however, these rates can differ significantly for different cadres, and these differences should be taken into account when further refining the HRH scaling-up plan.

Notes

1. It is important to highlight that, for Guinea and Sierra Leone, alternative numbers for current stock have been used in the existing analysis in the OneHealth Tool and BPEHS, respectively, which have not been used for this book.
2. For example, Liberia's Investment Plan report cites a 50 percent dropout rate from medical college.

Related Health Workforce Tables

TABLE B.3.1
Guinea: Trainees Needed Annually under Different Scenarios

Cadre	Scenario	2016	2017	2018	2019	2020	2021	2022	2023	2024
High-level cadres (doctors)	Base scenario	189	189	189	189	189	189	189	189	189
	Scenario 1	335	345	354	364	373	382	392	401	411
	Scenario 2	583	602	621	640	659	677	696	715	734
Mid-level cadres	Base scenario	300	349	410	488	576	680	805	952	1,126
	Scenario 1	532	619	727	863	1,018	1,201	1,420	1,678	1,984
	Scenario 2	924	1,077	1,264	1,500	1,769	2,087	2,467	2,915	3,446
Low-level cadres	Base scenario	208	210	386	234	248	272	302	335	377
	Scenario 1	513	527	798	592	624	672	730	794	873
	Scenario 2	930	956	1,417	1,076	1,134	1,219	1,321	1,434	1,572
Nurses	Base scenario	198	234	276	327	386	456	539	637	753
	Scenario 1	352	415	489	579	682	805	951	1,123	1,327
	Scenario 2	612	722	851	1,006	1,186	1,400	1,653	1,952	2,305
Midwives	Base scenario	98	116	137	163	193	227	269	318	376
	Scenario 1	164	195	232	278	330	390	464	550	652
	Scenario 2	282	337	401	480	571	675	803	953	1,129

TABLE B.3.2
Liberia: Trainees Needed Annually under Different Scenarios

Cadre	Scenario	2016	2017	2018	2019	2020	2021
High-level cadres (doctors)	Base scenario	31	31	31	31	31	31
	Scenario 1	53	55	56	58	59	61
	Scenario 2	92	95	98	101	104	107
Mid-level cadres	Base scenario	440	440	440	440	440	440
	Scenario 1	826	848	870	892	914	936
	Scenario 2	1,448	1,492	1,536	1,580	1,624	1,668
Low-level cadres	Base scenario	901	901	901	901	901	901
	Scenario 1	1,715	1,760	1,806	1,851	1,896	1,941
	Scenario 2	3,014	3,104	3,194	3,284	3,374	3,464
Nurses	Base scenario	197	197	197	197	197	197
	Scenario 1	414	423	433	443	453	463
	Scenario 2	736	756	775	795	815	834
Midwives	Base scenario	238	238	238	238	238	238
	Scenario 1	400	412	423	435	447	459
	Scenario 2	689	713	737	761	784	808

TABLE B.3.3
Sierra Leone: Trainees Needed Annually under Different Scenarios

Cadre	Scenario	2016	2017	2018	2019	2020	2021	2022	2023	2024	2025
High-level cadres (doctors)	Base scenario	47.1	47.1	47.1	47.1	47.1	47.1	47.1	47.1	47.1	47.1
	Scenario 1	81	84	86	89	91	93	96	98	100	103
	Scenario 2	141	146	151	155	160	165	169	174	179	184
Mid-level cadres	Base scenario	98	98	98	98	98	98	98	98	98	98
	Scenario 1	183	188	193	198	203	207	212	217	222	227
	Scenario 2	321	331	340	350	360	370	379	389	399	409
Low-level cadres	Base scenario	1,302	1,302	1,302	1,302	1,302	1,302	1,302	1,302	1,302	1,302
	Scenario 1	2,392	2,457	2,522	2,587	2,652	2,717	2,782	2,847	2,913	2,978
	Scenario 2	4,181	4,311	4,441	4,571	4,701	4,832	4,962	5,092	5,222	5,352
Nurses	Base scenario	64	64	64	64	64	64	64	64	64	64
	Scenario 1	117	120	123	127	130	133	136	139	143	146
	Scenario 2	205	211	217	224	230	237	243	249	256	262
Midwives	Base scenario	30	30	30	30	30	30	30	30	30	30
	Scenario 1	54	56	57	59	60	61	63	64	66	67
	Scenario 2	95	98	100	103	106	109	112	115	118	121

National Disease Surveillance

TABLE C.1
Scope of Country Profile Exercise

Component	Subcomponent	Feature
1. Surveillance and early warning	1.1. Case detection	1.1.1. Collection of information is done through routine surveillance. 1.1.2. Collection of information is done through community. 1.2.3. Collection of information is done through other event based surveillance.
	1.2. Reporting	1.2.1. Weekly and monthly reports are transmitted timely. 1.2.2. Disease outbreaks are reported timely.
	1.3. Verification	1.3.1. Reported public health events are timely verified and risks for populations are assessed. 1.3.2. Confirmed public health events are timely assessed.
	1.4. Data analysis	1.4.1. Data are analyzed on a regular basis. 1.4.2. Data are used for action.
	1.5. Feedback	1.5.1. Feedback mechanisms are present.
	1.6. Legislation	1.6.1. Legal context has been adapted to IHR requirements for surveillance.
	1.7. Coordination of surveillance	1.7.1. An operational national IHR focal point (IHR NFP) is in place. 1.7.2. Coordination of surveillance is clearly established. 1.7.3. Coordination for surveillance between human and animal health sectors is in place. 1.7.4. Coordination with the private sector is established. 1.7.5. Coordination between countries exists for public health surveillance.

table continues next page

TABLE C.1
Scope of Country Profile Exercise *(continued)*

Component	Subcomponent	Feature
	1.8. Resources for surveillance	1.8.1. Financial resources for surveillance activities are available. 1.8.2. Equipment and logistics are sufficient to conduct surveillance activities.
2. Strengthened laboratory capacity	2.1. Laboratory diagnostic and confirmation capacity	2.1.1. Laboratory services are available for diagnosis and confirmation.
	2.2. Laboratory networking system	2.2.1. Laboratories are a part of national, regional, or global laboratory network.
	2.3. Laboratory quality system	2.3.1. Measures to assure quality are in place
	2.4. Laboratory biosafety and biosecurity	2.4.1. Measures to assure biosafety and biosecurity in laboratories are in place.
	2.5. Coordination of laboratory	2.5.1. The central unit in charge of laboratory services is identified. 2.5.2. A mechanism to report laboratory results to the public health surveillance system is in place. 2.5.3. A mechanism to coordinate between human health laboratory and animal health laboratory is in place.
	2.6. Resources for laboratory	2.6.1. Resources for the contribution of laboratory services to surveillance are available.
3. Workforce training, deployment, and retention	3.1. Deployment and retention of surveillance staff	3.1.1. Human resources for surveillance are sufficient.
	3.2. Training for surveillance	3.2.1. Training needs are known. 3.2.2. Training capacities are in place.
4. Preparedness and response	4.1. Public health emergency preparedness	4.1.1. Plans and strategies have been developed and are in place.
	4.2. Rapid response capacity	4.2.1. Public health emergency response mechanisms are in place. 4.2.2. Rapid response teams are available.
	4.3. Coordination of rapid response	4.3.1. Coordination of response is clearly established.
	4.4. Resources for rapid response	4.4.1. Capacity to deploy resources during a public health emergency is present.

TABLE C.2
Summary of Results: Evidence on the Benefits and Impacts of Surveillance and Response Networks

Indicators / measures of value added	Case study network	Evidence of impact
Epidemiologic indicators		
Reduced time to detection	EAIDSNet	• Early detection of 4 Ebola outbreaks and points of transmission in Uganda
Cases/outbreaks averted	EAIDSNet	• Averted outbreaks and reduced cases of Ebola, Rift Valley Fever, Marburg, and wild polio virus
Effective early warning system with the capacity for trends assessment established	PPHSN	• Establishment of PacNet has resulted in the implementation of preventive measures against the spread of emerging and reemerging infectious diseases across countries in the region including dengue fever, influenza, measles, rubella, and SARS
Reduced time to action / effective response	EAIDSNet	• Reduced time of transmission of vital information from surveillance data for effective response
Magnitude of mortality and morbidity averted	EAIDSNet	• Containment of the spread of 4 recorded outbreaks of EVD in the region
Measure of disease risk factors for the development of early prevention interventions	MBDS	• Training of workforce on disease risk communication across countries in the Mekong Basin
Measures of improved International Health Regulations (2005) core capacities		
Increase in country technical capacity (including improved usage of ICT)	EAIDSNet; MBDS; SACIDS	• Successful pilot of a Web-based OneHealth portal for linking animal and human health disease surveillance (EAIDSNet) • Successfully partnered with University of Mahidol to trained cross-border officials on the use of Geographic Information Systems for research, outbreak investigations, and communication (MBDS) • Partnership with EAIDSNet on the pilot for a mobile phone-based system for rapid cross-border communication of animal-human health surveillance information (SACIDS)
Improved surveillance and usage of surveillance data for action / implementable policy formulation	EAIDSNet; MECIDS; PPHSN	• Improved framework for cross-border surveillance within the context of IHR (2005) and IDSR • Improved reporting system used for mitigating the impact of AI (MECIDS) • Streamlining of surveillance data across member countries
Improved preparedness and response capacity	EAIDSNet; MBDS; MECIDS	• Successful completion of a field simulation exercise in HPAI pandemic preparedness (EAIDSNet), including at the Kenyan-Ugandan border; • Successful preparation for and response to H5N1, dengue fever outbreaks, and natural disasters in Myanmar in 2008 (MBDS); • Successful preparedness and response to the H1N1 outbreak in the Middle East region (MECIDS)

table continues next page

TABLE C.2

Summary of Results: Evidence on the Benefits and Impacts of Surveillance and Response Networks *(continued)*

Indicators / measures of value added	Case study network	Evidence of impact
Number of cross-border sites established (points of entry)	EAIDSNet; MBDS	• Strengthened district health management teams at cross-border districts; • Expansion of cross-border sites from 4 to 24 in 3 years (MBDS)
Improved laboratory confirmation	EAIDSNet; across all regional networks	• Implementation of activities under the EAPHLN project to improve laboratory capacity in the region • Promotion of better laboratory practices and dissemination of standardized laboratory protocols
Appropriately trained and skilled human resources	EAIDSNet; MBDS; MECIDS	• Expansion of the HRH staffing capacity for disease surveillance and response using a OneHealth approach (EAIDSNet) • Improved capacity building for HRH: training of medical doctors in epidemiology and in disease surveillance and response (MBDS) • Development of common health workforce training protocols in core skill sets for member countries (MECIDS)
Health systems strengthening indicators		
Efficiency of an RDSR system	MBDS, MECIDS	• Improved cross-sectoral coordination for preparedness and response activities (MBDS) • Serves as an effective platform for countries to monitor emerging and reemerging infectious disease trends across member countries (MECIDS)
Improved coordination of disease prevention and control activities from community to national levels	EAIDSNet; SACIDS	• Establishment of Village Health Teams (VHTs) and reporting protocols to the district health information system • Serves as an effective bridge between the ministries of human health, livestock, and wildlife in the 14 SADC countries;
Allocation of resources during health planning	MBDS	• Allocation of resources for expansion of cross-border surveillance response sites
Improved country capacity in the health sector	EAIDSNet; SACIDS	• Institutionalization of a formal health unit within the East African Community • Serves as an effective bridge between the ministries of human health, livestock, and wildlife in the 14 SADC countries
Private sector engagement	PPSHN; SACIDS	• Establishment of PacNet

table continues next page

TABLE C.2

Summary of Results: Evidence on the Benefits and Impacts of Surveillance and Response Networks *(continued)*

Indicators / measures of value added	Case study network	Evidence of impact
Measures of multisectoral and regional cooperation		
Increase in cooperation among member states	MBDS; SACIDS	• Establishment of multisectoral border response teams (MBRTs) made of trained officials from member countries representing the health, animal, customs, and immigration sector (MBDS) • Effective surveillance of climate-dependent vector-borne disease with potential interspecies concern (SACIDS)
Joint outbreak investigations conducted	MBDS; EAIDSNet	• Joint dengue fever investigation by multisectoral cross-border response teams (health, customs, and immigration officials) between Lao and Thai provincial sites; joint typhoid investigation between Lao and Thai provincial sites; joint avian influenza investigation of cases in humans (MBDS); • Joint outbreak investigations for 4 EVD outbreaks

TABLE C.3

Essential Components and Activities under a Surveillance and Response Network

| | Country-level activities | | | Regional-level activities | |
| | | | | | |
Component	Community-based/ villages	District / local government (primary and intermediate public health care level)	National	Cross-border communities / villages	Cross-border districts	Transnational

Surveillance and information systems for early detection and analysis	• Routine and active / events-based surveillance (including at points of entry)
	• Training of community members for early warning, case detection, and rapid reporting to district health authorities
	• Sensitization and public awareness for livestock producers on animal diseases detection and reporting
	• Training on routine use of information and communications technology (ICT) for community-based surveillance and rapid reporting to district health authorities
	• Creation of an information sharing (mobile-based) social network
		• Active surveillance by district health workers (including at points of entry)
		• Capacity-building activities in surveillance and response (in animal and human health sector) for district health workers
		• Implementation of IDSR strategy
		• Implementation of other surveillance programs within the community and local government
			• Review and establishment of national priorities for infectious diseases affecting humans and animals
			• Linkage of community-based surveillance system to subnational (district) and national surveillance system (in real time)
			• Development of operational research protocols and sentinel surveillance capacity
			• Establishment of Sentinel surveillance pilot sites
			• Facilitate collaboration with the private sector for the development of a state-of-the-art surveillance data management, reporting, and communication system
				• Implementation / roll out of a *"basic package"* of surveillance activities at cross-border sites, including:
				  ○ Training of cross-border community workers for early warning, case detection, and rapid reporting to cross-border district health authorities
				  ○ Training on use of ICT for community-based surveillance and rapid reporting to cross-border district health authorities
					• Adoption of mobile-based platforms (mobile phones, tablets) for rapid cross-border coordination and sharing of animal-human health surveillance information in realtime
					• Rapid reporting of surveillance data to cross-border partners;
					• Regular cross-border meeting by district human health and animal health officers
					• Cooperation in animal movement border control
						• Development of harmonized reporting tools, and cross-border control protocols (including harmonized procedures for trans-boundary animal movement control)
						• Establishment of a regional ICT platform for efficient e-surveillance and incident management, and the use of Geographic Information Systems (GIS) to study diseases patterns
						• Link regional animal health information systems with OIE WAHIS and OIE-FAO-WHO GLEWS

table continues next page

TABLE C.3

Essential Components and Activities under a Surveillance and Response Network (continued)

Component	Country-level activities			Regional-level activities		
	Community-based/ villages	District / local government (primary and intermediate public health care level)	National	Cross-border communities / villages	Cross-border districts	Transnational
			• Development of incentives-based early reporting system • National Animal Diseases Information systems compatible with regional AHIS and OIE WAHIS and OIE-FAO-WHO GLEWS • Preparation of surveillance programs for a wide range of major diseases to inform the risk analysis process • Improved capacities for wild animal surveillance			• Training of health personnel including National IHR Focal points in participatory surveillance and early reporting of notifiable diseases constituting PHEICs • Development of an incentives-based mechanism to encourage early reporting of events as defined by the WHO and the OIE; and compensation mechanisms to encourage animal culling • Development of communication plans (including risk communication)

table continues next page

148

TABLE C.3
Essential Components and Activities under a Surveillance and Response Network *(continued)*

Component	Country-level activities			Regional-level activities		
	Community-based/villages	District / local government (primary and intermediate public health care level)	National	Cross-border communities / villages	Cross-border districts	Transnational
						• Strengthen technical and operational capacity of all actors involved in disease surveillance and response, including on cross-border cooperation for animal movement control, and rapid information sharing within the region • Design of an impact evaluation study to inform the prioritization of diseases, and to assess the value of an incentive-based approach to improving the functionality and effectiveness of a collaborative RDSR platform.

table continues next page

TABLE C.3

Essential Components and Activities under a Surveillance and Response Network *(continued)*

Component	Country-level activities			Regional-level activities	
	Community-based/ villages	District / local government (primary and intermediate public health care level)	National	Cross-border communities / villages	Cross-border districts
Strengthened laboratory capacity	• Capacity building for CHWs on early reporting of surveillance data to district health authorities, and to facilitate rapid laboratory classification and confirmation of suspected cases	• Implementation of quality assurance programs within district laboratory networks • Capacity building tailored to district health workers and laboratory personnel for early reporting and laboratory confirmation of cases • Innovative use of ICT to improve laboratory confirmation, including use of rapid diagnostic tests (RDTs) • Improvement of cold chain for vaccines / drug delivery	• Review, upgrade, and rationalization of laboratory systems (public health and veterinary public health) and development/ strengthening of national quality assurance programs • Strengthen laboratory data management system and its interoperability with the surveillance information systems • investments in RDTs and novel vaccine development (another area for private sector engagement) • Improve capacity of laboratories for active surveillance of antimicrobial resistance (AMR) and insecticide resistance	• Capacity building for cross-border CHWs on early reporting of surveillance data to cross-border district health authorities, and to facilitate rapid laboratory classification and confirmation of suspected cases	• Capacity building tailored to cross-border district health workers and laboratory personnel for early reporting and laboratory confirmation of cases

The Transnational column:
• Identification and strengthening of regional reference laboratories for priority infectious diseases
• Application of the WHO-AFRO Five-Step Accreditation process to accredit all laboratories in the proposed network to progressively meet the international certification with clearly defined parameters for turnaround time, quality, and proficiency

149

table continues next page

TABLE C.3

Essential Components and Activities under a Surveillance and Response Network *(continued)*

Component	Country-level activities			Regional-level activities		
	Community-based/ villages	District / local government (primary and intermediate public health care level)	National	Cross-border communities / villages	Cross-border districts	Transnational
			• Enhance laboratory systems with the capacities for real time biosurveillance of infectious diseases in humans and animals • Capacity building for clinicians on the use of surveillance data (from community to national levels) to improve case confirmation and diagnosis • Strengthen national veterinary laboratory services, based on the recommendations made from the OIE PVS evaluation and sub-sequent Gap Analysis, veterinary legislation review, and laboratory network improvement			• Partnership building with the private sector to support specific laboratory functions, such as the establishment of a specimen transporting network to facilitate the shipping of specimens within the region and internationally (to global reference laboratories) • Implementation of a regional quality assurance program and the development of common standards for national laboratories

table continues next page

TABLE C.3
Essential Components and Activities under a Surveillance and Response Network *(continued)*

Component	Country-level activities			Regional-level activities		
	Community-based/ villages	District / local government (primary and intermediate public health care level)	National	Cross-border communities / villages	Cross-border districts	Transnational
Pandemic preparedness and rapid response	• Community simulation exercises and drills in pandemic preparedness • Roll out of an Epidemic Control Toolkit[a] for community-based health workers (to be utilized at the household level) • Design of low-literacy, pictorial versions of communication tools; use of edutainment and other proven methods for improving interpersonal communication between community workers and household members to facilitate preparedness at household level	• Field simulation exercises covering activities in pandemic preparedness plans; • Management of vaccines, personal protective equipment procurement, and distribution logistics • Deployment of emergency response health workers • Establishment of designated health facilities for infection prevention and control (IPC) • Implementation of established IPC measures at the district and community levels	• Outsourcing of periodic independent monitoring and assessments of the core public health capacities of national structures to meet IHR (2005) and OIE Terrestrial Code; • Strengthen the delivery of IHR (2005) core public health capacities • Development/ update of National Pandemic Preparedness plans, Disaster Risk Management plans, IPC plans, standard operating procedures, and communication plans • Harmonization of pandemic preparedness plans into vertical disease control programs	• Simulation exercises and drills at cross-border communities and districts • Cooperation in joint outbreak investigations • implementation of activities under national and regional emergency response plans • Cooperation and support in the control of animals movements at cross-border sites • Awareness campaigns on rules/regulations related to animal movements at borders		• Tabletop, simulation exercises, and multi-country training on epidemiological investigations • Establishment of an evidence-based action plan and pandemic preparedness framework for the RDSR network • Establishment of cross-border sites and activities for cross-border cooperation; • Partnership building for multidisciplinary research on priority infectious diseases across other relevant sectors (agriculture, customs/ immigration, education and biosecurity) • Development of emergency response plans/tools

table continues next page

TABLE C.3
Essential Components and Activities under a Surveillance and Response Network *(continued)*

Component	Country-level activities			Regional-level activities		
	Community-based/villages	District / local government (primary and intermediate public health care level)	National	Cross-border communities / villages	Cross-border districts	Transnational
	• Develop effective mechanisms for distribution of IEC materials (including multihazard preparedness, emergency communication and advocacy tools, and safe hygiene practices)	• Surge capacity improvements • Establish mechanisms for improving access to, and enhanced delivery of, primary health care services for common illnesses. • Development of IEC and BCC tools tailored to district and local context • Training on regular test run of communication materials prior to an outbreak to promote education of priority issues and ensure local acceptance of contents.	• Establishment of a national emergency operation center / central hub for rapid response • Facilitate public-private partnership (PPP) to enhance supply chain distribution effectiveness during an emergency response • Support the establishment and involvement of private veterinarians in the provision of animal health services (incentives, equipment, enabling environment, • National capacity-building exercises on cross-border cooperation			• Support a regional epidemiological data bank • Use of GIS and other ICT tools to identify potential high-risk areas for disease outbreaks in the region • Regular analysis and use of national and subregional surveillance data to establish and implement rapid response activities • Set up of a contingency emergency response funding mechanism for swift mobilization and deployment of resources in response to major infectious disease outbreaks • Management of regional animal diseases vaccines banks

table continues next page

TABLE C.3

Essential Components and Activities under a Surveillance and Response Network *(continued)*

| Component | Country-level activities | | | Regional-level activities | |
	Community-based / villages	District / local government (primary and intermediate public health care level)	National	Cross-border communities / villages	Cross-border districts	Transnational
Trained workforce for deployment and retention	• Creation of a Volunteer Network: Rapid deployment of trained community-based health workforce (human and animal health) for routine surveillance during the delivery of primary health care needs at the household level • Strengthening of existing Community Animal Health Workers network, through: (i) improved regulatory and policy framework, (ii) registration, (iii) harmonization of curriculum and training, and (iv) supervision by veterinarians (public or private)	• Strengthening of local veterinary services through training on animal disease surveillance, control, and response; equipment availability (IT, office, etc.); and mobility means (vehicles, motorbikes, and operating costs. • Creation of a real-time database of alumni of the national FETP and FELTP for rapid deployment during an outbreak	• Establishment of rapid control measures to limit the domestic and international spread of disease outbreaks • Establishment of positions for field epidemiologists and laboratory specialists at the district level • Strengthen essential human resources for health (HRH) capacities for surveillance and response, and improve practices for the assignment and retention of skilled health personnel by strengthening capacities for HR management in line ministries	• Provide training, supervision, and other incentives-based mechanisms for community agents engaged in community-based surveillance and response for both public health and veterinary health • Deployment of community-based health workers (covering animal and human health) across borders	• Training in epidemiology capacity for cross-border district health workers (covering animal and human health)	• Development of harmonized procedures for transboundary animal movements control • Establishment/upgrade of regional collaborating centers (for animal and human health) to support national laboratories, research centers, public health institutes, and veterinary services • Support the development/upgrading of educational curriculums for training of country-level health workforce in surveillance and response for priority infectious diseases.

table continues next page

TABLE C.3
Essential Components and Activities under a Surveillance and Response Network *(continued)*

Component	Country-level activities			Regional-level activities		
	Community-based/ villages	**District / local government (primary and intermediate public health care level)**	**National**	**Cross-border communities / villages**	**Cross-border districts**	**Transnational**
	• Increasing the involvement of livestock farmers in the animal health system through awareness campaigns, training in best practices, support for their structuration in sanitary livestock farmers' organization- etc. • Supporting inter-sectoral interventions combining animal and human health service provisions within the community	• Management of a real-time database of emergency response public health and veterinary health workers ready for deployment • Promote the involvement of livestock farmers in the animal health system through awareness campaigns, training in best practices, and providing support to their structuration in sanitary livestock farmers' organization.				• Training of district- and national-level health workers in core skill sets, including training in data management, epidemiology and laboratory practices, risk analysis (including risk assessment, and risk communication, risk management), IPC, and case management of infectious patients and livestock • Establishment of education programs for veterinarians to graduate from regional Vet University (e.g., Dakar EISMV Dakar), to build good network for the future

table continues next page

TABLE C.3

Essential Components and Activities under a Surveillance and Response Network *(continued)*

Component	Country-level activities			Regional-level activities		
	Community-based/ villages	District / local government (primary and intermediate public health care level)	National	Cross-border communities / villages	Cross-border districts	Transnational
						• Promote joint HH and AH programs at the regional level including partnerships/twinning arrangements with international universities. • Identification of pools of experts in the region to support regional institutions, including the ECOWAS-WAHO and the RAHC, for planning and coordinating regional activities • Support the staffing of OneHealth centers in the region with highly qualified personnel.

Note: a. The Epidemic Preparedness Control toolkit is adopted from the WHO Humanitarian Pandemic Preparedness (H2P) project.

TABLE C.4
Pillars Related to Disease Surveillance and Response in Country Investment Plans

Priority pillar	Guinea Health Development Plan (2015–24)	Liberia Health System Strengthening Investment Plan	Sierra Leone Health Sector Recovery Plan
Priority area for improving epidemic, preparedness, surveillance, and response	Develop a health information system and health research	Strengthen epidemic preparedness, surveillance, and response, including the expansion of the established surveillance and early warning and response system to ensure it is comprehensive enough to detect and respond to future health threats	Improve the information system and surveillance for the implementation of the IHR (2005) core capacities
Costed item for achieving priority pillar	• Reorganize the NHIS by aligning drivers of subsystems health information • Strength integrated community-based surveillance and district health facilities for monitoring EVD and other diseases[a] • Improve the quality of health information • Improve the production, dissemination, and use of health information • Build human and financial resources, equipment, and infrastructures • Strengthen the institutional framework and coordination of research for health • Strengthen the capacity of research institutions for health	• Establish a National Public Health Institute, including a Public Health Capacity Building Centre and an Emergency Operations Centre, as core structures for the stewardship and implementation of the International Health Regulations (2005) • Establish Integrated Disease Surveillance and Response (IDSR) and Early Warning and Alert Response Network (EWARN) structures at national, county, district, and community levels • Set up comprehensive surveillance integrated data reporting and action frameworks • Improve capacity for public health laboratories (that is, build a national reference laboratory and four regional laboratories, upgrading one laboratory at Phebe Hospital to regional laboratory standards)	• Implement integrated disease surveillance and response systems (including Ebola) • Establish a functional national laboratory network with increased capacity of quality assessment, information system, and supervision • Strengthen health information system

Source: National investment plans.
a. Outlined under the Strategic Orientation pillar 1: strengthening the prevention and management of diseases and emergencies.

TABLE C.5

Cost Estimate for Implementing the Pillar on Disease Surveillance and Response under Country Investment Plans

U.S. dollars

Pillar	Guinea	Liberia (fiscal 2014/15 to fiscal 2021/22)	Sierra Leone (fiscal 2014/15 to fiscal 2020/21)
	Develop a health information system and health research	Develop an epidemic preparedness, surveillance, and response system	Strengthen the information and surveillance system
Base scenario	11,377,000	28,788,069	22,420,089
Scenario 1: Moderate case	11,377,000	58,902,543	22,420,089
Scenario 2: Best case	11,377,000	102,450,933	22,420,089

Source: National investment plans.

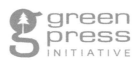